My Schizophrenic Life

My Schizophrenic Life

The Road To Recovery From Mental Illness

Sandra Yuen MacKay

Bridgeross Communications, Dundas, Ontario, Canada

Library and Archives Canada Cataloguing in Publication

MacKay, Sandra Yuen, 1965-
    My schizophrenic life : the road to recovery from mental illness / Sandra Yuen MacKay.

ISBN 978-0-9810037-9-5

    1. MacKay, Sandra Yuen, 1965-. 2. Schizophrenics-- Canada--Biography. 3. Schizophrenia. I. Title.

RC514.M312 2010   616.89'80092   C2010-905064-9

First Published in 2010 by Bridgeross Communications, Dundas, Ontario, Canada

ISBN 978-0-9810037-9-5

Advance Praise

VALUABLE LESSONS THAT MAY SAVE OTHERS

Sandra's autobiography offers a rare and sustained look into the challenges of living with schizophrenia. She lets us travel with her from the first early intrusions of paranoid delusions into her young teenage years to the long periods when the chaos of her illness dominated her life. She openly explores the ongoing challenges of coping with a mental illness and lets us witness her courageous and creative rebuilding of her life. Sandra's appreciation of the contributions of her steadfast family and many dedicated mental health workers is refreshing; seeing how much these efforts matter can help sustain families, friends and professionals during the painful ordeals that these disorders inflict on people. Sandra learns that, imperfect as they are, medications provide the foundation of her well-being; this is a valuable lesson that may save many others unnecessary anguish.

This important book should be read by anyone wanting to understand how someone can recover from schizophrenia.

Susan Inman, author of *After Her Brain Broke: Helping My Daughter Recover Her Sanity*, Vancouver, BC

COURAGEOUSLY TOLD, FAST PACED, INTERESTING AND READABLE

A fascinating perspective of growing up and developing a mental illness early in life, courageously told! Sandra MacKay has written a fast-paced, interesting and readable experience of learning to live with a complex mental illness; the more so with the dual aspects of a psychotic and mood disorder. She writes with keen insight so that the reader is part of the experience and learns from it simultaneously. The ongoing dialogue between Sandra, her family and her caregivers offers the reader a sense of the rollercoaster ride in dealing with the mental health system and shows also her transition to the road of recovery. This is an authentic and honest journey through an illness experience that teaches us the value of individual effort and the recovery process.

Sarah Sinanan, BA, BSc. OT
Coordinator, The Art Studios, Vancouver, BC

ARTICULATE, HONEST AND INSPIRING

A compelling and immensely interesting story of the author's journey to recovery after being diagnosed as a teenager with a serious mental illness. Sandra's insight and intelligence shines through in this well written exploration of the impact psychosis has had on her life. She recounts her experience in a way that allows the reader to understand and grasp the challenges of mental illness on an individual, family members, and friends. Sandra's story is articulate, honest, inspiring, and engaging - a 'must read' as it helps us to understand that people with mental illness are more than their diagnosis - they are people who, with tremendous courage, tackle the challenges and stigma of mental illness and show us that there is a path to recovery, to hope, and to realizing the meaning and purpose of one's own life.

Linda Proudfoot, B.Ed,
Regional Coordinator for Vancouver/Richmond, BC
Schizophrenia Society

HELPS US UNDERSTAND WHAT HAS SO LONG BEEN MISUNDERSTOOD

Society is indebted to people who are willing to talk about the experience of mental illness. I salute Sandra's story of her life so far. A life that includes recovery of herself, her purpose, creativity and voice. By listening to these lived stories we can understand the chaos and confusion of mental illness. It is through understanding that people can and do regain their health from mental illness that stigma can be reduced and eliminated. I admire and respect the honesty Sandra demonstrates to tell her story. She helps us to understand what has so long been misunderstood. I look forward to reading more chapters in her life.

Sandra Hale
Occupational Therapist
Clinical Assistant Professor, School of Occupational Science and Occupational Therapy, University of British Columbia

PUTS US IN HER SHOES

She writes very well with a great deal of insight and accuracy. She puts the reader nicely in her shoes experiencing the paranoia, misinterpretations, and hallucinations.

David Laing Dawson MD, FRCP (C)
Former professor of psychiatry, McMaster University, former chief of psychiatry, Hamilton Psychiatric Hospital
Author of *Schizophrenia in Focus*, *Relationship Management*, and *The Adolescent Owners Manual*

HOPE AND VITALITY

"My Schizophrenic Life" is a moving, powerful and informative story. Sandra MacKay sheds a brilliant ray of light on a subject that has long been kept in the dark. She promises and delivers hope and vitality – something that all too often eludes those who battle profound mental illness. I was very touched by this book and I commend the author for the brave soul that she is.

Merle Ginsburg
Program Coordinator
Consumer Initiative Fund
Vancouver Coastal Health Authority

A STORY OF TRIUMPH WITH LESSONS FOR ALL

There are precious few people who have experienced psychosis and can convey it accurately, clearly, and concisely. Sandra

MacKay's story is an important one for all of us in the mental health field -- doctors, patients, and their families. It is imperative that we take in the lessons she is imparting to us all, on how to manage, and in many ways, triumph, over chronic mental illness.

Julie Holland, MD author, *Weekends at Bellevue: Nine Years on the Night Shift at the Psych ER*. New York City, NY

REMARKABLY COMPELLING

While clumsily written and in dire need of a professional editor or perhaps even a ghostwriter, this volume is nonetheless remarkably compelling. The book takes on a life of its own as MacKay relates her lifelong struggles with severe mental illness. In particular, she illuminates the ways in which schizophrenic delusions can hijack one's life. MacKay vividly re-creates her world of schizophrenia, introducing readers to a whole new stratum of perception. Significantly, MacKay finds her salvation through art and writing, as she learns to capitalize on creative insights gleaned from her bouts with mental illness. **Verdict** MacKay's enlightening portrayal of her illness, hospitalizations, relationships, therapeutic activities, and quest for recovery will hold readers captive despite the elementary language and disjointed structure of the memoir. Like Kay Redfield Jamison's more eloquent *An Unquiet Mind: A Memoir of Moods and Madness*, this slight piece provides a surprisingly gripping narrative that will appeal to Jamison aficionados.

Lynne F. Maxwell, Villanova Univ. Sch. of Law Lib., PA

Table of Contents

Advance Praise...4

Foreword..10

Introduction...12

Early Signs of Impending Problems...............................14

Hallucinations and Delusions...24

Forced Hospitalization..36

Attempting A Return To School 52

From Rehospitalization to the Senior Prom....................67

Fighting Through School on Prescribed Drugs................83

The Challenge of Working...104

Wedding Bells..120

Dealing with Phobias and Deaths in the Family.............131

Relapse..142

Creativity, Coping, Strategies, and Ideations.................158

New Insights, Opportunities, and Sorrow......................168

Writing, Art, and Public Speaking.................................181

Stigma...197

Reflections..201

Biography..207

Foreword

What a timely and inspiring publication; an easy to read book that will attract those who know about mental illness and those who don't. It is easy enough for kids to understand, and is inspiring enough to engage experienced gurus. It certainly is a book not to be missed. *Toward Recovery and Well-Being: A Framework for a Mental Health Strategy for Canadians* is one of the important publications that will shape mental wellness of Canadians in the 2010s'. It speaks to two very important areas that our society has to face, promotes recovery for people living with mental illness, and reduces the stigma on mental illness. *My Schizophrenic Life: The Road To Recovery From Mental Illness* provides real life illustrations about recovery from mental illness and a candid understanding of mental illness, which de-mythicizes the stigma that goes with the illness.

This book beautifully captures Sandra's experiences and reflections along her journey to who she is today. In addition to narrating her personal story, Sandra also provides readers a comprehensive view of what mental illness is. Not hiding anything about mental illness and how the illness influences her daily life, Sandra powerfully speaks to the importance of hope and the recovery of mental illness. Her sharing also casts light on the importance of self, family, society and community in fostering hope and enabling recovery. It gives perspective to all of us on how we all should embrace such illness.

One of the advantages of writing a foreword is being one of the few people who can enjoy the book before everybody else does. I enjoyed reading Sandra's journey, her style of writing, and her courage to live daily life to the fullest. So dig in, and welcome to Sandra's journey of her heart, the term coined by Patricia Deegan. I hope you will enjoy this book as much as I did.

Michael Lee
Occupational Therapist, Certified Psychosocial
Rehabilitation Practitioner
Clinical Associate Professor, University of British Columbia

Introduction

If you have a relative, friend or acquaintance who has a mental illness, the insights in this book may inspire and help you. If you are unfamiliar with mental illness and want to learn more, other than hearing stories in the media about people who go off their medication, become drug addicts, commit suicide, or crimes against others, this book is for you too.

Life stories often start at the beginning but instead I'll start in the middle. I am in my forties, at the time of writing this book. Outwardly, I seem to be normal with a happy outlook and a smile on my face. I have a close-knit family and celebrate holidays and birthdays with them every year. My sisters, Penny and Ava, are both married with children and university educated. My father passed away at age 70, but he is still with me in many ways. I inherited his creative ability and drive to succeed. He was undaunted by stress and conflicts in his work, which led him to persevere and strive harder. My mother taught me independence and responsibility. I admire her generous and caring heart. Sometimes, I find it hard to live up to her expectations. Truthfully, she loves me despite my faults.

Despite my guise of normalcy, I don't have a so-called normal mind. I don't have visible disabilities but rather an invisible one. My current diagnosis is schizoaffective disorder, which includes a combination of schizophrenia and a mood disorder. My symptoms over the course of my illness have included paranoid and grandiose delusions, hallucinations, disorganized thinking, incoherent speech, and periods of mania and depression.

This is a true story about my journey of recovery from mental illness. I've tried to maintain accuracy and not veer from actual events. This is not meant as a diagnostic tool or a substitute for psychiatric advice. Some of the symptoms mentioned are unique to me. Most of the names have been changed to protect individual privacy.

Thank you to my family, friends and the mental health professionals who have helped me along the way. I thank fellow writers, Stuart Myers (Óchâni Lele), Jayne Gale, Cleveland W. Gibson and Susan Inman for their support. I also thank Marvin Ross of Bridgeross Communications, my publisher, and the people who took the time to read my book and write blurbs.

Some excerpts in the book were taken from my articles, which originally appeared in *The Bulletin*, a mental health magazine published by the West Coast Mental Health Network. They have been edited from the original.

Early Signs of Impending Problems

September 1965 - December 1979

The disturbed mind lives in a world that intersects with common reality. Stimuli may trigger symptoms, which magnify into psychosis. The unreal becomes real. The brain is possessed, flowing with fear and anguish, and the future is clouded with uncertainty.

My mental illness came as a surprise to our unsuspecting family. We had few skeletons in our closet. Mental illness was never mentioned in our family history even though it can be passed on through the genes.

In Vancouver, British Columbia, my family lived in a white stucco house with blue-grey trim in a quiet neighborhood with many kids my age. My sisters and I jumped on the trampoline next door. I taught myself to swim at a friend's pool during a sweltering August. I got into trouble like any other kid, but also enjoyed making people laugh at my jokes.

I was proud to be the lead in a Christmas play in grade seven. We acted out "The Twelve Days of Christmas" with some added funny lines. I was the receiver of the gifts. The more I received, the angrier I became. At the end, I sent away the bearer of the gifts and a male teacher came forward, offered me a long-stemmed red rose and led me off the stage to great applause.

When I entered high school, however, my introverted tendency and feelings of inadequacy expanded exponentially. In grade eight, I had a locker between two boys' lockers. The lockers were newly painted with warm, bright colors. Mine was mandarin orange. I nicknamed the boys "Mutt and Jeff" because one was short and the other was tall. I rarely spoke to them other than offering a soft hello.

"Would you like to get together after school?" Blair asked. He was the taller of the two, blond and blue-eyed.

"Ah, no. I have to study." I buried my head in my locker and reached for my grey knapsack.

"We could do that."

"No, I don't think I can right now."

"Well, if you ever change your mind, just let me know."

I was flattered, but too anxious and doubtful to say yes. It was easier to shut people out than become vulnerable.

One day towards the end of term, Mutt and Jeff serenaded me with Carole King's song "You've Got a Friend." I was moved that they sang to me. After they left, I slung on my knapsack and walked home with a spring in my step.

I resembled the characters in *The Wizard of Oz*: a scarecrow without a brain, a tin woodman robbed of emotions, a lion with no courage, and Dorothy, lost in a foreign land. In the story, the wizard recognized that the first three needed faith to overcome their problems; likewise, I didn't believe in myself either.

In high school, I was one of the top students, but I was also one of the shyest, quietest, and most awkward teenagers anyone could meet. I hid behind my glasses and had braces to correct crooked teeth and an overbite. The orthodontist had me wear headgear fourteen hours a day with elastics on my teeth.

I was shorter than most of the other girls my age and very thin. I envied the way my friends got along with male students. I buried my head and rarely said a word to anybody. I never volunteered answers in class.

At a friend's birthday party in the summer of 1979, just before I turned fourteen, a group of us danced to slow music in her basement lit by candles and Japanese paper lanterns. I was terrified to dance with a boy a year older than me. It wasn't so much his age, but he was about a foot taller than me.

"What's your name?" he asked. I froze. "I said, 'What's your name?'"

I bit my lip and looked down at the brown shag carpet. I envisioned myself sinking into the rug, melting like a Popsicle, until I disappeared. I tilted my head away from his gaze and refused to make eye contact.

"Didn't we meet before?" he said.

"Ah, no. It wasn't me."

"You were out cycling with your friends this summer," he persisted. "Your gang stopped by my house to say hello. Don't you remember?"

I shook my head. I stepped back, confused. He walked away and shook his head, leaving me to sink into the carpet alone.

I blushed with embarrassment because I behaved so ineptly. Later on, I vaguely recalled cycling by his place but it was too late to say anything to him.

It was during this time that I began to experience symptoms of apathy, an inability to engage socially, a sense of aloneness, mental confusion, and problems with attention span, which brought me closer to developing psychosis. To most, these behaviors could be interpreted as normal teenage problems. Thus it would have been hard for anyone to guess the turn my life was about to take.

#

When I started grade nine in September of 1979, I was eager. I liked school because I had keen interest in many subjects. I'd already chosen my locker on the main level near my friends' lockers. I knew they'd all be there ahead of me. I always slept in until the last moment, dressed, grabbed a slice of raisin toast with butter, and rushed out the door with my knapsack.

I was already thinking about field hockey. I played on the school team in grade eight and looked forward to playing again. I liked the uniform in the school colors burgundy and blue. The top was powder blue and the skirt was a plaid kilt. We even got bloomers and matching socks to wear. Cleats, a field hockey stick, shin pads and a mouth guard completed the outfit. I enjoyed playing halfback, aiding defense and passing to the forwards. Players on the team got out of class early to get to the games on time, which made me feel special.

I lived about ten blocks from school. In a superstitious manner, I avoided stepping on the cracks in the sidewalk. On the way to school, I always cut through the lanes and the same dog would bark at me. I never saw the dog as it was hidden behind a six-foot cedar fence so I didn't know its size, but I was determined not to change my route because of it. I had a right to walk down that lane any day of the week. That was the extent of my courage in those days.

17

Repeatedly, I smelled a strong odor of vinegar in one particular lane. It was so strong that I held my nose when I passed.

One weekend in early September, I slept over at Candice's house in Burnaby. Candice was a year younger but we were friends. I brought my purple sleeping bag and slept on a mattress on the hardwood floor. I slept in late and woke up alone in her bedroom in the basement. I heard voices talking from the direction of a bedroom upstairs.

"Is she staying another night?" The voice sounded faint.

"I don't know," answered another voice. "I don't want her to stay. Let's get rid of her."

Distressed, I thought I had overheard Candice's mother and sister talking about me. I got dressed and went up to the kitchen. The smell of coffee brewing made my nose wrinkle. My friend and her brother sat at the breakfast table, eating toast and jam and making funny hand gestures. I thought they were making fun of me. Did they all want me to leave?

So, that's how it began. I smelled a strong odor in the lane and I heard voices talking about me.

These early warning signs most of us would dismiss by trying to form logical answers to them. Maybe it was the smell of rotting food in the trash. Maybe I could hear through the vents in my friend's house because the house was quiet. In retrospect, I believe these events were olfactory and auditory hallucinations, the first signs of my break with reality.

#

I had a crush on several boys at different times in

18

school. I rarely conversed with them, but rather admired them from afar.

Truthfully, I was too nervous and immature to have a relationship with a boy. I had only kissed a boy once on a dare. I wished I could make small talk or have a conversation that lasted more than a few minutes with boys or girls at school but I couldn't.

When I talked to my sisters, we joked but rarely talked about emotions. If people asked me how I was feeling, I said that I was fine, instead of revealing my unhappiness or loneliness. The problem was I didn't really identify with anyone. No one could pierce my shell of isolation, which shielded my sensitive nature.

Because of my mother's upbringing, she wasn't too forthcoming with advice or information about the facts of life or dating. Her parents had an arranged marriage and came from China. My maternal grandmother, whom I called Po Po in Cantonese, had false papers stating she was born in Victoria, British Columbia. Years later, the federal government offered amnesty to anyone who had come to Canada illegally during that time. My Po Po wanted to come forward, but my maternal grandfather, whom I called Gung Gung, disagreed. "Let sleeping dogs lie. You don't have to tell anyone. Don't worry."

My grandmother didn't speak much English but she got by. When she was angry or excited, she switched to Cantonese. I couldn't understand or speak Cantonese or Mandarin. Instead I'd wait for her to settle down and convert back to English. I doubt she told my mother much about dating either.

I talked with my mom in the bathroom while she

was putting on her make-up. We had only one bathroom in our house, with a folding door to separate the two sinks from the toilet and bathtub.

"When will I be ready to date?" Would my parents let me if someone asked me? I needed boundaries. I wanted to know if there was a curfew I needed to follow.

"That's up to you, isn't it?" She applied a red hue to her lips and put the lipstick back in the drawer. She walked away without another word.

I would have benefited greatly from a frank discussion or advice about the physical, hormonal and psychological changes that I was experiencing. I had no idea of my parents' expectations or ways to handle social situations. I knew drugs and alcohol could be harmful, but I wasn't given a set of rules. Instead, I had no guidance.

I talked to some of my friends who recalled that their mothers didn't explain much about the facts of life either. They laughed.

"Ask Penny," they said. I would have asked my older sister Penny, but I didn't know exactly the questions to ask.

My mother relied on Sunday school and the Bible to teach her three daughters about moral behavior. I developed a strong conscience. I was meek, polite and extremely humble. When I bumped into someone in the hall at school, I mumbled an apology even if it wasn't my fault.

#

The buzz of loud chatter and laughter filled the crowded halls of my school before and after classes. I quietly made my way down the corridors with my head down, trying not to be noticed. I didn't gossip much, but I was sure other students were spreading rumors about me.

"Michael wants to ask Sandra to the Christmas dance," whispered a girl in math class.

"What's he waiting for?" asked another student.

"I don't know."

Michael was on the basketball team. In math class, I'd call across the room, "Hey, Mike, what did you get on the test?"

"Seventy-eight percent. What did you get?"

"Only ninety-eight." I grinned. Math was one area I was confident in and that allowed me to brag a little. I was shy, however, when it came to asking him to sign my annual.

So when I heard rumors he was interested in asking me to the Christmas dance, I clammed up. I went into shy mode. I didn't talk to him and never let him see when I was looking at him. He sat in the front row in one of my classes and would sneak a look at me. I'd turn my head and focus on the window or straight in front of me. I was afraid and unable to respond to him. I didn't want to communicate because it would make me vulnerable, or lead to teasing or embarrassment.

I thought the other students were laughing at me and whispering behind my back. They called me "four eyes" or "ugly duckling" or say "she's so dumb she can't even talk." One of the students shoved me in the halls. "Get out of the way, loser," he said.

Ashamed, I hunched over until my chin was lower than my shoulders, giving me the posture of an old lady with a humpback. The rumors and name-calling disturbed me. I went through the robotic motions of attending class but interacted with others less and less. My fragile nature didn't allow anyone to get close to me.

"Did you hear any rumors about me at school?" I asked a friend. "I think people are saying things about me."

She shook her head. "No, of course not."

Even though she denied it, I remained unsure.

Michael never did ask me to the Christmas dance. I thought no other boys at school would ever ask me out after that. I thought it was my fault because I withdrew into myself and didn't speak up. I was a little mouse scurrying along, too timid to be able to spend time with a boy or anyone. Feelings of rejection and disappointment rose inside of me.

#

I became extremely depressed that winter. The days grew short. My sisters and I slept in the living room by the Christmas tree on Christmas Eve, hoping to catch Santa filling our stockings. Truthfully, we wanted to catch our father or mother in the act. They were pretty sneaky about it.

We awoke Christmas morning to see freshly fallen snow outside. We enjoyed opening our presents and laughed together. We dressed and got ready to go to my grandparents' home for Christmas lunch. My Po Po was a great cook. I never saw her use a recipe or measuring spoons or cups, but she could cook the best Chinese food I ever ate. I opened the front door and saw Taylor on his bicycle at the edge of our sidewalk.

Taylor was my square-dancing partner in phys ed class. I was very surprised to see him at 11 A.M. on

Christmas morning. I waved and smiled and he did the same. I thought it was such a strange coincidence.

During Christmas vacation, I was outside in the front yard when I saw two figures at the bottom of the street. I heard one boy say, "There she is. Hide."

"She can't see us from here," the other boy replied.

It did not occur to me that they were too far away to be heard. I heard the voices as clearly as if they were speaking right next to me.

My sister Penny and I decided to walk downtown from our house. It was a long way but we could window-shop and have lunch downtown. We started on our way. I thought I heard the boys' voices over the sounds of the traffic even though I couldn't see them. When we crossed the Granville Street Bridge, I saw two figures following us. One wore white pants. I wondered if they were tailing us. I thought one of them might be Taylor.

"Does anything seem odd to you?" I asked Penny. "Do you think we are being followed?"

"No. Are you trying to scare me?" she said. I shook my head. I didn't say anything else, but continued to look back with worried glances.

By the time we got downtown, I couldn't hear or see anyone following us.

The voices I heard were real to me. Logically, it's impossible to hear people talking at normal volume from sixty yards away on a busy street or bridge. It was like I was in a vacuum where I could hear things very acutely. I thought I had super-hearing like a comic book hero.

Hallucinations and Delusions

January 1980 - September 1980

I went downstairs to our new recreation room in the basement. It was very large with couches, a ping-pong table and a television. There were two windows but they had no curtains. I heard Penny talking as I entered the room.

"Who are you talking to?" I asked.

"No one."

I looked at the open window and saw a flash of someone outside. I thought a trespasser saw me and ran off. I saw him run past another basement window, through the backyard and out to the lane. I couldn't make out who it was but suspected it was Taylor.

"Who was that?"

"I didn't see anyone," she said.

Wasn't she just talking to the person in the window? Something was amiss. I thought perhaps my eyes were playing tricks on me. Penny had no reason to lie.

Later, I was alone downstairs playing solitaire, sitting cross-legged on the cream carpet. I heard murmurs from the window. I looked up but couldn't see anyone in the darkness outside. Then there were two voices. I thought one was Taylor and the other was Darren.

The real Darren was a student at school. He was popular, with a good sense of humor, and flirted with the girls. Darren was tall with dark hair, like a typical love interest in a romance novel. He lived a few blocks away. I thought perhaps he knew Taylor from school and Taylor had asked him to come.

First, I was annoyed, thinking they were trespassing on private property. I just ignored them, hoping they'd lose interest and leave. There wasn't much to see in our basement.

"Can she see us?" said the voice of Darren.

"I think she's ignoring us. Let's go," answered another voice, which I thought must be Taylor's. I looked toward the window with curiosity.

"Shh. She's looking at us."

I wasn't fond of Taylor, but Darren interested me. He knew Michael and could connect me with the in crowd. If I became his friend, he might introduce me to his other friends and maybe I could become as popular as well. I stared up at the window and winked.

"She winked at me," I heard the voice of Darren say. "She knows we're here."

"No way," said the other voice.

"I'm positive she did." The voices faded away.

I was excited that boys were paying attention to me but also I knew it was wrong for them to spy on me through the window. Conflicted, I was unsure how to deal with the situation. I turned off the television and went upstairs.

Later that week, we were eating dinner, when I heard sounds coming from outside the kitchen window. By this time, I'd heard voices outside briefly for the last three evenings after dark. I could picture them crouching around the house and listening, hidden by the bushes and darkness. I tired of them and wanted them to leave.

"Dad, there are people outside the window. They're listening to our conversations and watching us at night."

Certainly, my father would get them to leave. He would protect me.

"Don't lie. No one's out there," said my younger sister Ava. She was nine. She reached for her glass and spilled milk on the table. Mother wiped it up with a napkin.

"She thinks a boy is following her because she's got a crush," said Penny, eyeing me.

"No, I don't." I stuck out my tongue.

"You told me you had a secret admirer." She put a forkful of rice in her mouth. I didn't remember saying anything to her but maybe I had.

"Eat your dinner," my mother said.

I looked forlornly at my father. He was more occupied with his meeting that evening than dealing with my concerns. I doubted if he even heard me. I took a bite of broccoli. The soy sauce tasted salty in my mouth. I ate the rest of my meal in silence.

After dinner, I went downstairs and turned on the TV. No sounds came from the window, but I sensed someone was there.

Discouraged and uncertain about how to handle the nightly visitors, I did nothing. I didn't contact the school or talk to Darren or Taylor directly. Inexperienced and unable to solve the problem, I allowed the intrusion to continue.

I developed a relationship with the voice of Darren. I sensed he was angry because I had tattled on him. I developed a rapport with this omniscient presence and he paid more attention to me than to anyone else. He watched and listened to things I did or said which made me feel special. But my affections wore thin because he was still a trespasser. Sometimes I could hear other voices outside as well.

The more I was drawn to Darren, the more I withdrew from my family and friends at school. My curiosity and attraction to this fellow student metamorphosed into a magnetic pull I couldn't resist. Obsessed with him, I went to his house to confront him one evening. I wanted the spying to stop. I wanted to see the real Darren face-to-face.

An older man answered the door. "May I help you?"

"I'm here to see Darren." I wondered if the man was his father.

"What for?"

"To sign my annual." I lied, keeping my hands behind my back hidden from view.

"What's your name?"

I told him my name and he called for Darren.

Seconds later, Darren appeared, carrying his annual. "Who are you?"

"Sandra."

"How do I know you?" He looked deadly serious. How could he not know me after watching me for weeks?

"From school."

"How can I help you?"

"I want to know why you and your friends keep bothering me." My eyes narrowed in an icy glare.

"Who?"

"Oh, Taylor, Larry, Marsha and Cole." I was sure I recognized the other voices as well.

He frowned. "I don't know those people."

"This has been going on too long and I want it to stop!" My temper rose another notch.

"How long has it been?"

Was he mocking me? "Three weeks," I replied.

"I'm sorry I can't help you."

"This isn't over. I'll get you back!" I shouted. Suddenly, I despised him. I ran down the stairs and back home. He lied to protect himself and his friends, I thought.

When I look back now, I realize the world I built around him was false. He wasn't attracted to me. He wasn't trespassing or spending his evenings spying on me. He was a stranger.

The voices continued to bother me but at different times of day. I'd hear whispers on the bus, to the point I thought someone was hanging on the back of the bus, hitching a free ride. I wondered why the other passengers couldn't hear the voices. I heard voices through the ventilation system at school and I'd miss out on verbal exchanges during class. I had difficulty following lessons. I'd hear voices in the car that seemed to come from the radio speakers. When I walked to school, I could hear shouting over the sounds of the traffic.

One day, as I was riding my bike, I heard multiple voices yelling loudly, "Fireball, fireball! She's a fireball!" I turned but saw no one except in the cars driving past on the busy street. I pedaled faster, but I couldn't escape the shouting. I sped down a long hill without holding the handlebars. The cool wind blew on my face and my heartbeat quickened. In exhilaration, I felt I could take flight.

Other times, the voices turned on me and called me names. I heard six at a time, calling me "geezer" or "jackass." The voices were all around me, making my head spin. Mortified, I fell into an abyss of depression that opened up beneath me. I was spiraling down unable to save myself.

I only showered in the morning when it was daylight and the spies weren't there. I thought they could see me on the toilet in the evenings if they stood on each others' shoulders and peeked through the bathroom window. Mortified, I could hear them laughing outside. I dressed in the dark so they couldn't see me between the curtains. I felt shame that if I told my father, he would punish me for allowing them to spy on all of us and keeping it a secret. I was unable to think rationally or ask for help.

My parents must have been concerned about my behavior, but they passed it off as a teenage phase. I bathed less. I'd wear the same clothes everyday. When my mother greeted me in the morning, I'd ignore her. I believed they were in denial that anything serious could be wrong with me because I still managed to get good grades and do my chores.

My mother took me to our family doctor to ask about my lack of response. She thought I had a hearing problem. The doctor took a tuning fork and attempted to test my hearing. I could hear its sound; however, I was distracted and refused to respond to the doctor's questions.

"She doesn't have a hearing problem. She has attention deficit disorder," he said. His diagnosis was a gross error. Still my parents didn't understand the seriousness of my condition.

The voices became infrequent and subsided after eight months, but I still suspected others were watching me. I believed my parents were in contact with my peers. I thought they were punishing me and that I was a victim of a series of cruel jokes.

I believed there were microphones and cameras built into the walls of my house because the voices always seemed to know which TV show I was watching or my location inside the house. I felt eyes on me wherever I went.

One night, I thought raw eggs were being thrown at the window. Afraid to open the curtain, I hid under the covers and cried myself to sleep.

The next morning, I looked out the window and there was no evidence of eggshells, but only beads of condensation on the glass from a cool night.

I once enjoyed food immensely but now everything I ate tasted bland. I forgot which day it was.

I welcomed the first precious minutes upon waking, which was the only time my mind was clear of foreign thoughts. By the time I dressed and ate breakfast, the fear and confusion took hold once again.

#

September arrived which meant I was back at school, enrolled in grade ten. A year had passed since my peculiar experiences began. I was deeply immersed in a psychotic state, but no one knew the severity of the problem. It had remained undiscovered for a year. When one is under that type of pressure, however, a break is inevitable.

After dinner, I routinely washed the dishes and cleaned up the kitchen. It usually took me an hour to clear the counter, empty and load the dishwasher, scrub the pots and pans, and dry the hand-washed dishes.

I had a habit of listening to music with headphones

on. I'd sing along at the top of my lungs and dance. Singing loudly was my defense to shut out my invisible aggressors. Foreign thoughts still entered my mind. I thought I recognized my cousins' voices singing on my records. I also thought my peers were communicating to me through the lyrics of the songs. After dinner, I put on the headphones and started to tune everyone else out. I turned the volume high and sang. My father came into the living room.

"Go wash the dishes," he ordered.

I sang in his face and shouted the lyrics.

"Go clean up."

I said no and gave him a look. He slapped me soundly across the face. I was surprised but also felt very hurt and angry.

"Hit me. Hit me again! Come on, you want to hit me," I retaliated.

"Go to your room."

"No, I'm supposed to wash the frigging dishes. Isn't that what you want? Isn't that the only thing you want from me?" I yelled. He didn't care about me. In my perceptions, he was in the enemy camp.

He put on his shoes and coat and walked out the door. My mother said that he had a meeting but my impression was that he walked out on me.

I never forgave him for slapping me. My parents spanked me when I was younger, but for him to slap me across the face at age fifteen I felt was very wrong.

"Why did you do it, dad?" I asked later.

"It wasn't what you said. It was the way you looked at me."

"What kind of look was it?"

"It was evil," he answered. "Sheer evil."

Horrified, I thought he hated the evil he saw in me enough to strike me. But where did this evil come from? I wasn't a sinful person; I was innocent. I felt resentful and hurt, and thus I distanced myself from others even more.

I cleaned up the dishes, contemplating smashing all the plates on the floor and poisoning the leftover food with cleansing powder as a form of revenge. Ava offered to help wash the dishes, but I told her to go watch TV. I wanted to be alone even if the chores took longer.

I went out to the lane. I sat on the gravel leaning against the wooden fence, pounding it with my fist. It was starting to get dark. I walked aimlessly up the lane and away from the house. As I walked to my elementary school five blocks away, I talked to myself louder and louder. I walked around the empty schoolyard. I saw a sedan parked on the side of the road. I thought I saw Taylor in the backseat. Was he tailing me? How did he know where I was?

I walked to the other side of the school and up the steps to the main entrance. I pounded on the door with my fists, shouting, "Come get me, you bastards! I'll get you in the end. I'll hunt you down until the day I die."

I wailed until I couldn't cry anymore. "Kill me why don't you!"

"Who's there?" I heard a voice call out.

Afraid of being caught for creating a public disturbance, I raced down the steps and returned home. When I got back to the house the sky was dark. My mother had some friends over and they were talking and laughing in the living room. I went into the kitchen, but it seemed different somehow. I had an eerie feeling that a psychic force was there in the kitchen. I checked the cupboards but nothing was amiss. It was the strangest feeling of a presence haunting me in the room. Was I possessed by the devil? Or was God punishing me for being born a sinner? I wanted to blame someone so I blamed my parents. I needed to make them pay.

My tormented mind overloaded. I felt chills in my back. My fingers were like ice and my hands started to shake.

I walked into the bathroom and flicked on the light. The first thing I saw was a tube of toothpaste. I grabbed it and squeezed the contents onto the sink, counter, mirror, bathtub, windowsill and curtains.

I went downstairs to the recreation room and grabbed my favorite deck of cards. I ripped the cards to pieces, leaving a trail from the front door, to my dad's car parked in front of our property. I even shoved some down the open sunroof of his car. By destroying them, I erased the memory of happy hours I had playing card games. After purging my pain, I quietly went to bed.

Early the next morning, half-awake I overheard my father on the phone. "Kevin is in charge now," he said.

I took this to mean that a classmate named Kevin was leading the plot against me and my father knew about it.

When I got up later, my family had already left for school and work. I went into the bathroom. There was no sign of toothpaste anywhere. I went outside and saw the playing cards had been taken away. All the evidence was gone. I was stunned no one in the family said anything to me. They covered it up like it never happened. How could they not respond? What was happening in my family that they ignored my behavior?

Feeling betrayed and desperate, that evening I took a bottle of Indian ink and a paintbrush from the basement. I opened the front door. Penny had recently painted the floor of the front porch with a pale blue-grey hue. I dipped the brush in the ink and wrote block letters across the porch, which read, "Who are you and why are you doing this to me?"

When I opened the door the next morning, the black paint had been wiped away leaving black smears all over the porch floor. Everyone had left the house, leaving me alone. I was distressed but I still went to school that day.

Penny found me standing outside the drama theater, waiting for class to start. "What's the matter with you?" She looked very troubled.

"Nothing. What's the matter with you?" I retorted.

"Do you know about the ink on the porch?"

"Yes, I did it. The toothpaste too."

"Why are you doing these bad things? I told mom and dad I was worried. Do you hate dad?"

"No."

"Do you hate me?" she asked.

I shook my head.

"Why did you paint the porch?"

"Because I was angry."

"I'm going to tell them something's got to be done. We can't go on like this."

I opened the door to the drama theater. I looked back but she was gone.

When I got home, I turned on the stereo and put on the headphones. My mother returned from work and turned off the stereo.

"We have to talk," she said. "I want to know why you're getting out of control. When Dad saw the message, he thought it was from someone he worked with. He never thought it could be you. You broke his heart."

"I want answers."

"Do you blame us because we're not home enough?"

"I need you to care about me!"

"Of course we care about you."

"You hate me. You all hate me."

She looked at me with hurt in her eyes. I stared back with defiance.

I felt utterly alone. Slowly, the gate was closing separating me from a normal existence, but I didn't realize it. I internalized my emotions until I exploded in destructive behavior.

Sometimes one wishes to turn the clock back. We regret past events or wish we could change the past. I wished that my painful experiences could have been erased. Instead, they haunted me for decades. I could not separate truth from fiction.

Forced Hospitalization

October 1980 - January 1981

One afternoon in the kitchen, I studied a recipe from a cookbook. The kitchen faced south. Its pale yellow walls were brightened by the sunlight. In the spring, daffodils would bloom in the backyard, and in the summer, wild raspberries grew in the garden.

That day, I wasn't concerned about the garden. I was absorbed in my first attempt to make peach cobbler. I made a mistake in the recipe, adding the flour too soon. As I was preparing the dish, my mother came into the kitchen, carrying a bottle of pills.

"Sandra, take these pills." She held out two white pills.

"I don't want to take those. I don't know what they are."

"They'll help you."

I refused. She left the kitchen.

I heard a knock at the front door. My mother answered. Murmurs followed. The door separating the kitchen from the dining room opened and a man in a white uniform entered.

"Hello, how are you?" He smiled.

I was surprised. "Fine."

"We want to take you down to the hospital."

I imagined that he was ready to take me away in a straightjacket to a white padded cell. Certainly this only happened in movies. I grinned at the thought. "Why?"

"You need to go there now." He was firm.

I didn't object. He led me from the kitchen to an ambulance waiting outside. For some reason, I wasn't afraid but calm. I didn't argue. I was sure he could overpower me if I resisted.

Perhaps now someone would listen to me. I got into the back of the ambulance with him while the driver, also dressed in a pressed, white uniform, put the ambulance in gear.

"I've never been in an ambulance before," I said. "Are you going to turn on the siren?"

"No siren on this trip."

"Why are you taking me there?"

Instead of answering my question, he asked me my name, age and other details. "What day is it today?"

"Saturday." I looked at my sneakers.

"Who's the Prime Minister of Canada?"

"Pierre Trudeau."

"What does it mean to not 'rock the boat'?"

I thought he was kidding me. "Do you think I'm rocking the boat?" I jested.

"Answer the question."

"It means don't make trouble." I figured the series of questions were designed to measure my lucidity.

He wrote something on his notepad. He checked his watch. We rode the rest of the way in silence.

The emergency room at the hospital was busy and crowded. I was told to wait for my mother who arrived in a separate car with an elder from the church. They sat there with long faces as if the world was ending. I didn't realize the depth of my mental problems.

I thought perhaps this was all a game or setup and

soon Darren would pop up and yell, "Fooled you!" Certainly, if he came clean this huge mess could be sorted out. I desperately needed to talk to him because he could explain the real story or so I falsely believed.

Restlessly, I paced, did jumping jacks and pretended to skip with an invisible rope. We waited for over two hours. I was called into a room to be assessed. A male doctor and a nurse talked to me first. He asked me a battery of questions. "Why are you here?"

"Because I'm a wonderful person," I said. My flippancy was a defense against others. Because of my manic state, I spoke inappropriately. I reacted based on feelings of fear and intimidation.

He gave me a disapproving look.

"My father slapped me."

"That's not why you're here."

"Isn't that abuse?" I countered.

"Are you experiencing anything?"

"Like what? School?" He waited for my next answer. "They're following me. They're trying to bring me down."

"Who are they?"

"Students from school."

"What are their names?"

I reeled off four or five names including Darren.

"What are they doing?"

"Causing trouble. Making my life miserable. They're out to get me." My tension was so high that I felt like there was a bomb ready to go off.

"Do you feel in jeopardy?"

"Yes!"

"Do you want to harm yourself or others?"

38

"I want to kill someone." I reacted with aggression and anger. In truth, I didn't want to hurt anybody but verbally lashing out was a defense mechanism.

"Have you used LSD, crack or any other drugs?"

"No!"

"Roll up your sleeve," said the nurse. She checked my arm for needle marks. The doctor and nurse were doing a routine check but I knew I wasn't an addict. They left and another doctor came in and asked more questions.

Then the first two doctors and a third talked to me again. I repeated the story again. Each time I told the story, I became more uncertain. I became more vague about details and unable to explain my experience in a logical fashion. I was tired after waiting so long. Four hours after arriving in emergency, I was admitted to a children's ward.

"Do you want to say goodbye to your mother?"

I refused. My stomach growled. "Got anything to eat?"

At that time, there was no separate psychiatric ward for teenagers at that hospital. I didn't know the other children's diagnoses or reasons why they were there. The ward had dull green walls and the windows were barred. There was a kitchen area with a large table for eating. An adjacent room had a television and stereo system. The carpet was old. I was put in a room with another girl who was very nearsighted. I could tell because when she read, she held the book two inches from her nose. We gathered for dinner. The food was brought in on a trolley and heated up in the kitchen if needed. I seemed to be the oldest in the group. The others looked no older than twelve.

After dinner, we watched a movie then were told to

wash up and get ready for bed. They gave me hospital pajamas to wear. The sheets were well worn covered by a thin, white, woven blanket. The pillow was too flat to give much comfort.

I fell asleep without tears for the first time in a long while. I felt protected from peering eyes that I had experienced previously.

My aunt came to visit me. She brought in some knitting. As she sat there, she worked on a jacket with a Navaho design.

"I wish I could knit," I said.

"Here I'll show you."

After some practice, I could do a knit or purl, but I kept losing stitches. She put her knitting away.

"Why am I here?" The doctors and nurses had told me nothing.

"You have paranoid schizophrenia."

"What's that?"

"You'd know better than me," she smiled.

"When will I get out of here?"

"When they decide you are well enough to leave."

"I don't want to fall behind. What shall I do?" Of all things, I was worried most about missing school.

"Listen to the doctor and don't forget your medication."

"What medication?"

"For Pete's sake! You're on Haldol. You're on injections," she exclaimed.

I remembered vaguely being poked with a needle for blood tests routinely given to all patients, but I was so out of touch that I didn't know they'd given me an injection.

I still had no concept of the severity of my condition. The label "paranoid schizophrenia" didn't mean much to me at this point. I needed more information about my illness but instead no one really talked to me in depth about schizophrenia.

I met with a psychiatrist on the ward. Her name was Dr. White. She looked more like a hippie than a doctor with her long flowing skirts, sandals and mane of curly hair. When she smiled, small wrinkles would form at the corners of her eyes. Despite her pleasant demeanor, I was hesitant at first to share any information with her. She had the power to keep me in the hospital.

"How are you doing?" she asked.

"As well as can be expected. It's alright here, but I really need to get back to things."

"What things?"

"Oh, school, university, career, my life." The small room suddenly felt smaller. I lost track of time. I wondered how long I'd been in hospital. It seemed like weeks.

"And if you can't fit in and don't finish school, what then?" she asked.

"I refuse to believe this is the end of the road. None of the nurses or even you had the courage to tell me I have schizophrenia. Why is that?"

"Paranoid schizophrenia," she corrected. "You wouldn't believe it even if you wanted to."

"What do you mean?" I implored.

"You don't have the capacity to understand. Do you want to see your mother?"

"Not really." I looked down at the floor. I felt indifferent to my family and the doctor as well, but my mood was unstable. I could lash out at any time.

"She wants to see you."

I nodded. She went to the door and my mother entered with tissues in hand. Her eyes were red and swollen. Her nose was red.

"Allergies, mom?"

"I'm crying for you," she said.

I looked at Dr. White. "Why is she crying? She brought me here. Isn't that what she wanted?"

"You're seriously ill. You may not know it, but you're ill," said Dr. White.

"Sandra, I love you," said my mother.

Suddenly, I felt a jolt of anger and confusion. How could she love me? I swore at the top of my lungs. "You're destroying my life! You're all crazier than me. Let me out of this prison. No one talks to me. No one helps me."

My mother cried and cried. I began to wail and scream. The room seemed to expand and contract. I felt an invisible force push down on me so I couldn't move from my chair.

I couldn't explain to the doctor my bizarre thoughts at the time. Instead, she only saw the outbursts and aggression.

Two nurses hauled me out of the office and took me to a quiet room where they gave me a sedative. The walls were cream with no windows. A dim light gave the room a soft glow. There were no objects in the room except a mattress. I fell asleep on a mattress on the floor. Later, I awoke. I tried the doorknob and it was unlocked. I stepped into the hall and a nurse escorted me back to my room on the ward.

I had no understanding of my mother's feelings at that point. I didn't recognize the degree to which I had hurt her. The visit had cost her a lot emotionally. Instead, I was preoccupied with my own thoughts and feelings. My mother wasn't there for the next session with Dr. White.

By the next day, with my mother gone, I settled down. A woman who worked in the unit asked me if I would complete an IQ test. I'd never had an IQ test and agreed.

There wasn't much to do on the ward. I wasn't interested in reading books or writing.

After several days, I was getting antsy. I really wanted to get out of that bleak, depressing ward. I felt restless and wanted to escape. One night, I went to bed with my day clothes on and sneaked down the hall and out of the ward. Elated, I chuckled to myself about how easy it was to get away. I was free but I needed a place to sleep. I walked a mile and a half to home. I found the key under the backdoor mat where it was always hidden. I entered my house, crawled into my bed, and fell asleep.

In the morning, I heard the phone ring in the kitchen. My father answered then hung up. "She's missing from the hospital. She's been missing since last night."

I overheard my mother say, "Why didn't they call us sooner?"

"I'm here." I came out of the bedroom half-awake and rubbed my eyes.

Mom and Dad looked at me with a combination of relief and concern in their eyes. They kept their distance so as not to agitate me, knowing I might react or lash out. "Why did you run away?"

"I don't want to be on the ward. It's monotonous. You're cut off and you can't go anywhere. I can't play the stereo loud or listen to my music." I didn't trust my parents fully but it was better at home than in the ward.

After a discussion between my parents and the psychiatrist, they decided I would stay home as an outpatient and not leave the house unsupervised. My mother refused to let me listen to loud music, stating it would overstimulate me. I was given medication that put me to sleep for most of the day. The full dosage was too strong, so under the doctor's directions, my mother split the pills, cutting the dosage significantly, and gave me half or a quarter tablet four times a day. My condition didn't improve. As the days progressed, I complained about the pills because they blocked out my memory and made me foggy-headed.

My parents and I didn't talk about my symptoms. My mother was unprepared for the day-to-day care of a mentally ill daughter. She had no psychiatric training but made sure I took my medication. I complained constantly about drowsiness, restlessness and a sore throat, which were side effects of the medication. At times I spoke incoherently. I didn't even know the name of my prescribed medicine. I didn't make any progress at home. My mother took time off work to care for me but soon my parents decided I needed more help.

My parents took me for a drive. I was glad to get out of the house. We arrived at an adult psychiatric unit at the University Hospital. My first impression was that it was roomy, comfortable and remarkably quiet. The carpet had a geometric pattern and the walls were tinted with warm tones. There were no bars on the windows this time. I thought we were only visiting but I soon realized their intention was to admit me.

"No, I'm not staying here," I said to one of the staff when my parents were out of the room. I felt cornered and angry.

The psychiatric nurse folded his arms and said to me, "As parents they can admit you. We have your medical report, stating you are mentally ill."

"What about my rights?"

"Once you are admitted you cannot leave until you are well enough."

I demanded to speak to my father. He came into the room. "How dare you double-cross me? How could you put me in this nuthouse?"

"You have daggers in your eyes. Are they for me?" He looked very sad and weary. "Why the hostility?"

"You have no idea," I said. "My life is over."

My parents left. I had no choice but to stay. The nurse returned with a waiver I was to sign.

"Can you explain the waiver?"

"It simply states you turn over your rights and agree to be treated in this facility."

"What if I want to leave and escape?"

"We'll pick you up and bring you back."

I hesitated. If I signed this waiver, I might be signing my life away. What if it had a hidden clause?

"You'll be better off if you sign it." The nurse folded his arms. He grew impatient. "Sign it now."

I felt intimidated, so I gave in and signed the waiver.

A fellow on the ward showed me around. He was

short and wore a turquoise shirt. He seemed to be around nineteen or so but I didn't ask his age. He was a patient as well. There were private and semi-private rooms in the ward. Two rooms were locked at all times. The locked rooms were for patients who potentially could harm themselves or others. I stayed away from that area but I could hear the patients shouting. There was a lounge, large dining area, television, laundry room and a meeting room. There was one payphone.

Escorted to another part of the hospital, I was given an electroencephalogram to check for any abnormalities in my brain. They used a sticky substance to attach the sensors to my head.

"Can I have a copy of the printout? Can you explain it to me?" I was curious, wondering about the results of the EEG.

"I need you to fall asleep," said the no-nonsense technician. "We need to chart how your brain behaves when you are asleep. Take this." She gave me a paper cup with pink gel inside.

"I can't drink this!"

She forced it to my lips and I swallowed it. "Close your eyes and try to sleep."

I closed my eyes but I had rapid eye movement caused by anxiety. The technician put her hand over my eyelids to calm my eye movement.

After twenty minutes, an attendant roused me and ushered me in a wheelchair back to the ward. I never got to see the printout.

#

What does one look forward to while staying in a

psychiatric ward? Not much. Days passed, blurring into one another. I spent a lot of time pacing the halls or dancing in the music room. Patients shuffled around talking to themselves with shaky, jerky movements caused by medications. Others chain-smoked, staring off into space or talking to themselves.

We went on outings along the trails around the university campus where the hospital was located. We also visited the botanical gardens. The leader of our group smoked a pipe. He reminded me of Raymond Burr. We walked through the Nitobe Memorial Garden. A guide talked about the religious and philosophical significance of the design. "Each stone, shrub or tree in the garden is placed in a certain way to create harmony."

I walked around the garden. I felt a sense of peace I hadn't felt for a long time. It was good to be outside and breathe fresh air surrounded by nature. I felt free from my inner demons for the first time in a long while. The change in environment released me from the pressures I faced at school. My paranoia had diminished. I had no hallucinations in the hospital.

We also visited the swimming pool and a gym. I was glad to get some exercise after being cooped up in a ward most of the time. In the gym, we played volleyball. One of the fellows picked me up and carried me when our side won. We cheered. I smiled and laughed. My mood had changed. A year before, I was so withdrawn that no one could get near me. On the ward, I came out of that shell enough to socialize with the others. I think my new openness was a result of feeling safe in hospital. I didn't talk a lot, but I laughed and listened to the others.

47

One of the nurses invited me to play a game of chess.

"Oh, I'm not that good at chess." I knew the rules but seldom played.

"It's for fun. C'mon, let's play."

I wasn't good at advanced planning strategies. In chess, I was unable to think several moves ahead and anticipate the moves of my opponent. I played offensively, but soon moved my chess pieces without forethought. The game turned in his favor and he won in the end.

"I'm glad I lasted as long as I did," I remarked.

"You played well."

I shook my head.

"I mean it, you did play well," he said.

I wasn't one to take compliments well. My perfectionism didn't allow me to feel good about myself. I denied myself satisfaction and didn't accept approval from others. This personality trait suppressed growth in self-confidence, which hindered me from maturing along the same path as my peers. Joy in life isn't easy when one doesn't like oneself.

The food on the ward was surprisingly good including seafood on puff pastry, roast beef, turkey, chicken and mashed potatoes. Breakfast was toast, eggs and bacon, pancakes or French toast.

In the cafeteria between meals, a lot of the patients smoked. "Here have one," offered Jason, one of the men on the ward. I guessed he was in his early twenties.

I took one out of his pack and he lit it with a match.

"You don't know how to inhale," he said, chuckling to himself.

"Yes, I do." Not willing to admit otherwise, I took a

long drag. I coughed so hard that tears came to my eyes.

He laughed at me. I made a face and put out the cigarette.

During the day, I spent a lot of time in the music room, listening to albums. One day, I was listening to The Rolling Stones. Jason came in and sat beside me. He pointed to the door. "Lock it."

"Why?" I didn't move from my seat.

"We're going to get it on."

He proceeded to touch and caress me with one hand. I was curious and I let him. I was flattered he was attracted to me. I didn't really know if it was wrong to allow him to touch me. I was naïve and vulnerable to his advances. My mother never taught me ways to handle such situations. My own common sense was flawed.

The fellow in the turquoise shirt came in. Jason pulled his hand away from me. The fellow left. Jason stood up and locked the door. He resumed his former seat, closed his eyes and continued the sensual touching.

A moment later, a staff member called from outside the door. "Open up. You've got a minor in there."

I looked at Jason. He looked at the door. We didn't move.

"Okay, we're coming in." The nurses unlocked the door and we were hauled out.

I figured Jason didn't know I was only fifteen because it was an adult ward. I thought I was equally responsible. I didn't object or try to stop him. It didn't really mean anything to me, I told myself. I denied I was harmed in any way. I didn't hear anything from the staff about the incident.

The next day, I saw him kiss a woman on the ward. He definitely considered himself a Don Juan. I ignored him for a while. He lost interest in me.

The doctors tested me on several medications, trying to find one or a combination that helped me the most. I fainted in the hall. They put me on a stretcher and checked my heart. I don't know why I fainted, but maybe it was stress-related or due to numerous medication changes.

They gave me another IQ test. It took a lot of concentration and energy to answer all the questions. Later, I asked a psychiatrist about the results. She said that I scored above average and had superior intelligence according to the tests at both hospitals ranking in the 95 to 97th percentile. Some say IQ tests don't mean much. Other factors in a person's life affect his or her ability to succeed. I thought it was significant, that despite my psychosis, I did as well as I did.

Although I was academically smart, it didn't mean I could flick a switch to cure my illness.

The doctors said there is no correlation between one's level of intelligence and schizophrenia.

In the years to follow, however, I lost some of my ability to remember, reason and concentrate because of the volume of excess information I processed daily. My obsessions and false ideas on top of my schoolwork and daily activities put my brain into overload. I had a difficult time memorizing facts, words and images, and writing essays. Some of my learning ability was diminished by the medication too. It was hard for me to learn through listening. I had trouble organizing my thoughts when taking notes in class. If the illness didn't cause enough problems, the side effects from the medication did. The pills made me drowsy and lethargic, affecting my alertness.

After another two months in hospital, Christmas arrived. I was allowed to leave the ward to celebrate Christmas with my family. They were happy to have me home overnight. My troubling thoughts had lessened. I was stabilized on Loxapine. A month later, one of the psychiatrists in charge of my case said that I could go home soon. I felt better than I had over the past year, but apprehensive about adjusting to the outside world.

Attempting A Return To School

February 1981 - August 1981

I was discharged under the care of Dr. White. I had requested her because she seemed more empathetic than the male psychiatrists I had met. I think it was partly because she was a woman and I desperately needed someone who would understand my difficulties as a young female, my attraction to the opposite sex, and my lack of ability to socialize with my peers. I returned to high school on a cold, wet January morning. My school counselor made it possible for me to continue in the regular school term despite missing three months.

I saw Dr. White, twice a week at an outpatient clinic. She was one person I could talk to freely about my illness.

"Why didn't anyone help me sooner? I was ill for a year before anyone did anything."

"Sometimes families are in denial. They don't want to believe anything is wrong. They ignore problems they fear or don't understand. You hid your illness for a long time. Could you have asked for help?" said Dr. White.

"I did and no one answered me."

"Painting words on the porch isn't the proper way to ask for help. You acted out without thinking about the consequences. You damaged private property."

I disliked her criticism. How could she not understand? "I was at the end of my rope. It was bound to come out some way or another. Don't you understand the stress and confusion I had at that time? What else could I have done? How else would my illness have been discovered?" I wanted empathy not judgment.

"You should have talked to your parents or a school counselor."

"I did try to say something to my father. I told him the curtains didn't close properly leaving a gap. I needed them fixed because people could see inside my bedroom."

"What did he say?"

"He said, 'Why would anyone want to watch you?' Another time I said something at dinner but no one listened. Am I to blame because they were blind to my behavior?"

"Most people in your situation would have checked it out or done something about it."

"It's fine for you to say that now. But if you were I, you would have dealt with it the same way. I was traumatized." I changed the topic. "I feel like a freak. I think all the students know I'm ill. All day long I think the words, 'They know. They know.' Darren is in my French class. I think he's sending his thoughts to me and can read my mind."

"How could that be possible?" she challenged.

I ignored the question. She believed it was illogical, but wasn't telepathy possible? What if I had a brain wave frequency that others could access? "Maybe things would improve if I changed schools."

"It would be the same. You'd still have the paranoia."

"I think they're out to get me." I had read a little about schizophrenia. Suffering from delusions, paranoia and emotional imbalance, I had all the classic symptoms of mental illness. Suspicion that people were plotting against me was also a symptom. Intellectually, I knew certain beliefs were part of the illness but they fooled me. Each false thought was a new interpretation or addition to my growing obsessions. I felt compelled to figure out where the dividing line between truth and illness lay. I lost concentration and changed the topic again. "The other students are so bright. I don't think I can keep up in class."

"Try your best. Do you need a tutor?"

I stopped talking and stared at a crack in the wall.

"What are you thinking about?" she said.

"Nothing." I had segments of time when I would blank out and just sit and stare. Sometimes this happened during lunch hour at school or during sessions with Dr. White.

Sometimes I felt like I was in a tunnel where there were no clues to direct me - just blackness. The tunnel held all my experiences, past and present, real and psychotic, in my consciousness. I lived in a web of falsehoods, linking events together that had no logical connection. I lost track of time and place.

I stared at a crack in the ceiling or at the carpet motionlessly. Eventually, I focused and came back to the present.

"I wish I was over twenty."

"Why?" asked Dr. White.

"Then I'd be over all this. I wouldn't have to live like this."

"You know mental illness can be chronic."

"Don't tell me that! I don't want to live like this forever."

I joined a group for troubled teens. We met after

school once a week with a nurse and social worker. I could identify with the sense of social isolation the other youths experienced. We talked about appropriate behavior and the difficulties of neglect and abuse.

By April, my mind seemed to clear. It was like the confusion that had caused me so much grief was gone. My mood lifted. The symptoms seemed to have subsided. I was no longer occupied by paranoid thoughts pounding in my head. I seemed to be handling my school courses and functioning better at home.

Dr. White stopped the medication, thinking perhaps it was a singular psychotic episode and not a chronic case. I breathed a sigh of relief. Two weeks later, however, my accelerating, distracted thinking returned and I needed to go back onto Loxapine.

Because of my first remission, as short as it was, I knew sanity. I saw the disturbed thinking as outside of reality. Since then, I had the hope of recovery.

The first insight I had was to acknowledge my illness and recognize the importance of taking medication. Without my daily dosage, I knew I would relapse. Secondly, I knew if I had any side effects or worsening of symptoms to alert someone right away, either a family member or a mental health professional. Otherwise, my symptoms would go unchecked. I learned to be honest and upfront in order to identify the problem and get help when needed. Sometimes one hopes for the best and is disappointed. Sometimes one hopes for a better life, but it doesn't go that way. Sometimes one tries so hard to live a normal life, to succeed in school or career, and to fit in, but the path is not clear-cut.

For some reason, I thought I had enough energy, motivation and hope that I could conquer my illness. As a teenager, I wanted to succeed in all areas of my life. I wanted to surpass others and was full of ambition. Perhaps, my dreams of the future were foolish, considering I had a disabling illness, but I was pigheaded enough to try.

#

Mania may cause hypersensitivity to sights, smells and sounds like a high without drugs.

When I had my headphones on, my endorphins would multiply. I'd dance and sing to the songs of The Rolling Stones, Led Zeppelin, or Queen.

One day after school, a layer of freshly fallen snow graced the streets and sidewalks. I danced in the streets, singing a song. My shoes left imprints in the snow on the road. A group of ladies having a tea party gathered at a window and watched as I danced past, waving and smiling.

Psychosis is deceptive. It slips into the conscious mind, drawing one into an alternate world. The line between reality and dreams bends and blurs. My delusions became concrete beliefs I could not shake. They seduced me into believing I had supernatural powers to know the past and future, and read other people's minds. I also believed I had the power to telepathically communicate to other people which was amplified by radio waves. So if I had the radio on at night, I believed my thoughts would broadcast over the radio to others.

Living in psychosis was ten times more exciting than reality. Being the center of the universe in my fantasies was something I craved because it fed my ego and put me in a manic state. Inside I was still a fearful child with an inferiority complex. By believing I was a genius with fantastic abilities was much more desirable than a reality of unhappiness, boredom and disappointment.

Dr. White told me about a technique to stop intrusive thinking called "stop therapy." One should shout out or think the word "stop" when one sensed one's mind starting to go in the wrong direction. Now if I were on the bus or in class, do I really want to yell out "Stop"?

Stop therapy never worked for me because basically I didn't want the delusions to leave. The thinking was part of me. The voice of Darren was my only contact when others neglected me. The invention of Darren filled the void I experienced at that time.

I didn't want the euphoria to go away. It was almost as if I brought it on voluntarily, addicted to my own mania. But in the end, as pointed out to me, I paid every time I went into that other world. It distanced me from others, got me off track, and left me feeling low. Sometimes it took weeks to level out and reach some sort of temporary equilibrium until the next wave.

Manic episodes were short-lived. One day I'd be on top of the world in my grandiose delusions, and the next day I'd come down, feeling self-pity. I wish I could calm down gradually, take a nap and everything would be fine. Instead, I would crash and burn like a plane out of control. After each cycle of mania and depression, I felt depleted and slept for hours.

Even positive experiences could cause stress. I would come home tired after a busy day, burst into tears and cry hysterically for an hour.

I grieved every bad thing that happened to me. I blamed others and myself for my misfortune. I believed others continued to play tricks on me and block my attempts to succeed or better myself.

I'd think about my relationship with the voices and the deep sense of guilt that I allowed the invasion to continue as long as it did. I was ashamed and felt a loss. I was convinced the voices belonged to real people. I felt their scorn. I regretted the fact I hadn't gone for help sooner.

Blaming others wasn't good because it created a major conflict in my already tenuous relationships. If I vocalized my distrust and anger, it only led to problems at home. Blaming myself led to destructive emotions.

"Dad," I said, one day on the back porch, "If I killed myself, would you be happier?"

"That's not a thing to ask," scolded my mother.

"I'd never forgive myself." My father sighed and shuffled into the house. He couldn't handle emotional conversations. He rarely opened up about his own fears around my illness and unknown future. It hurt him to see me fall into bouts of depression or hysteria, but he never told me. Penny told me how much he cared, years later after he passed away. Ava was only nine when I got ill and didn't really understand the extent of my psychosis.

Penny remained on the porch beside me. She whispered, "I can't bear the idea of you hurting yourself. Don't do it." She hugged me. Her eyes welled up with tears.

I felt like Sisyphus punished in the Underworld, pushing a rock up a hill. No matter how hard he pushed, the rock would roll back down the hill and he'd have to start over. I struggled with the same issues over and over, always falling into the same emotional traps. And so, the cycle continued for a long time.

#

In therapy sessions, I communicated my fears and dreams to Dr. White. "What would my life be like without illness?" I asked her.

"You'd still have some of the same issues you have now."

"What do you mean?"

"Come out of yourself. Talk, make friends, be a person."

"Are you saying I'm not a person?"

"Act normal and share your feelings."

"That's ludicrous. You have no idea how hard it is. Act normal is your best advice?"

She redirected. "Are you going to go to the spring dance?"

"The what?"

"If you want to feel included, participate in some extracurricular activities."

"No one will dance with me."

"Ask someone."

"Can't do it." I raised my hands in protest. "Everyone despises me. I might as well have leprosy."

Sometimes she'd encourage me but other times she would just calmly listen. Discussions with her about my negative feelings and thoughts allowed temporary relief week to week. Sometimes, when I felt overwhelmed with sadness, talking about my worries and disappointments only reinforced my distress.

Medications prevented the severity of my symptoms but didn't block them out entirely. If the dosage was increased too much, side effects were more apparent, interfering with my ability to carry out daily tasks.

On another visit, I sat in Dr. White's new office. She had relocated her office to a building next to the university campus. They ran a day program for outpatients there. Her office was small but had a window. From where I sat on a couch, I could see the blue sky and trees in the back of the property. The room was dim and the air was cool. I fiddled with my hair and bit my fingernails. A roll of toilet paper sat on the table in front of me in case I started to cry.

"I saw The Rolling Stones on the psych ward. They were there," I said.

"That's your belief, but it's not true," she said.

"How do you know? You weren't there."

She shook her head in dismay.

"I tell you I saw them," I countered.

"I'm sorry you feel that way."

"I don't need your condescending attitude. I tell you I met famous singers, musicians and actors."

"Sandra, you're taking this too far. Why would they be there in the hospital?" She knew she wasn't getting anywhere with me.

"I must have written notes asking them to come."

"Why would they come?" she argued.

"Because I'm a songwriter." I fidgeted with my hands.

"Oh, really. What do you write? Do you play an

instrument?"

"No, I can't read music."

"Yet, you can write songs?" she asked.

"Yes, I write lyrics by singing into a microphone. I hear my songs on the radio. I'm famous but in secret."

"You're living in a dream world," she contested. "You're building yourself up but really it's wrong. Try to understand that the things you believe aren't true."

"No one understands. Aren't you here to help me?" I pleaded.

"I understand but I can't say you're right. It's not part of common reality. Your experiences are different from others." She tried so hard to reason with me. "What's the alternative if these experiences aren't real? It doesn't make you a bad person."

"When I think that way, I feel invulnerable. If I throw away all the dreams, it means my life is worthless and I suffered for no reason."

Truthfully, I felt violated because I thought people were controlling my mind and watching me constantly. I was grasping onto straws, trying to find a way to prove my problems were someone else's fault. I didn't want to face the stigma that I was ill or feel self-blame that I had brought the illness on myself.

" Schizophrenia is a brain disease. It isn't the fault of the individual or caused by a weakness in the person."

"Why me? Maybe it's all true."

"Sometimes you have to leave the sinking ship for the lifeboat." She wanted me to let go but I couldn't.

"The lifeboat can tip. I could drown in the current." I shifted my position in my chair. I was restless from the medication.

"These things you cling too will only give you more pain." Dr. White knew I hung onto my beliefs like a lifeline.

Sometimes the things I said didn't make much sense but helped me to purge my pent-up emotions.

"Darren is using psychological warfare against me. I hate him but I love him. He's the worst and the best. I'm so in love I can't stand it."

"Slow down. You're not making sense. Listen to your words." Again my thinking was confused and she knew it.

"Michael grins at me when I walk down the school corridor. He thinks I'm a big joke."

"What did you do today?" She wanted me to stop rambling.

"I can't understand the French teacher. She gives the instructions in French. I don't know when the tests are coming or which pages to read."

"Practice your French."

"I can't speak it either. I have no one who will practice with me. Michael and Darren are in that class. I feel so ashamed I can't keep up. I spend the whole class looking straight at them."

"It's impolite to stare."

"They don't care who I am or what I do. I stand out like a sore thumb. They must know I'm crazy."

#

As my illness progressed, my delusions grew larger and more complex. My symptoms no longer consisted only of a few unexplained events but encompassed my whole life.

I suspected I was adopted and that my parents didn't really love me. I developed a fascination with celebrities. I thought I met famous people in hospital. The man with the pipe, who looked like Raymond Burr, became him in my mind.

I developed a false belief structure based on similarities of appearance of other people. I would be listening to a record with the headphones on and stare at the picture of the singer on the album cover. Through some trick of the mind, I'd make a connection between the singer and someone I met in the past. The likenesses were so similar between the singer and the person I met that I would believe I met famous celebrities.

Objectively, the doubles I perceived were invented by my mind. I believed my psychiatrist was an imposter and part of the plot. My imagination soared, putting me over the edge. I no longer lived in the present but was more concerned with the past and future.

Everything related to Darren, a series of mysterious notes I wrote which contained the answers to my dilemma, an altered childhood, and an unsolved crime of conspiracy. With a supposed photographic memory, I could see the past and relive events. I built numerous stories in my head to explain reasons why things happened to me.

In my artificial world, everyone and everything were interconnected. I projected false memories or associations with the past, linking events in my life like a row of dominoes. Each domino or single false memory was part of a complex network of deception against me. I predicted future outcomes. I'd look for signs like the time on my clock. If it read eleven minutes after eleven that was

63

significant to me. I believed at certain times, a wormhole or channel would open up and link the present to a specific time and place in the past or future.

If my psychiatrist disagreed with me on a particular point, I'd challenge her. It was like a game of chess, each of us putting forth our best offense and defense. No matter what she said, I defended my position. Every time she made a point, I'd counter it with a circular argument. I'd say anything to hang onto my grandiose delusions because if they were true, it meant I was important and in control. The truth was I was out of control.

Looking back, I can also see the pattern of the way that the illness evolved. Depression, social isolation and insecurity made me open to having an imaginary friend. The belief that I was a genius or had supernatural powers was the answer to feelings of inferiority. The worse I felt about myself, the more welcome the grandiose delusions became.

#

Outwardly, I didn't behave like the other kids at school. My movements were stiff or exaggerated because of my medication. When someone did make an effort to speak to me, I didn't respond in a normal fashion. I had difficulty with small talk. Most of the time I was too preoccupied with my thoughts that I couldn't put sentences together. I desired to reconnect with my peers.

My solution was to be candid. I told some of the students at school my exact diagnosis, just in case they wanted to know. I ran into Janice after school.

"Where have you been? I haven't seen you for months." Janice looked concerned.

"Oh, I was in the hospital. I have paranoid schizophrenia." I said it casually, as if I'd been away at camp.

"What? Are you joking?" She looked shocked.

I shook my head.

"Well, it's good to have you back. Sorry, I've got to run."

I told some of my other acquaintances, hoping they'd show sympathy. I tried humor as a way to connect.

"Hi, Al. Would you like to hear a secret?"

"Not really."

"I escaped from the funny farm. I'm a bona fide psycho." I grinned.

"I don't want to continue this conversation. Stay away from my locker."

I think my expectation was that people would pat me on the back and say, "You did it! You got through it and now you're back on track. Good work, Sandra!"

To be back at school was a personal triumph, considering the fears I had of certain fellow classmates and my constant ineptitude at conversing or retaining instructions in class. Was it too much to ask that my peers would recognize my ability to persevere and rise above my condition? But no one said much other than "See you later" or "Don't call me."

I was making progress, doing well in school, opening up to others, rekindling bonds with my family, and gaining some confidence. I still did my chores. My parents expected me to work hard and deal with my issues with my doctor.

I kept striving. My goals were always about the next

step or challenge to gain recognition and approval. I rarely reflected on my development as a person. I couldn't depend on others. I had to make it on my own.

The medication slowed me down. I had trouble in phys ed class and on the field hockey team. I couldn't keep up with the speed of the game or run 400 meters without huffing and puffing. I felt bloated and tired constantly. I slept a lot. Afraid of gaining weight, I went on a diet and lost twelve pounds. I had a waffle for breakfast with a dab of syrup. Lunch was a bowl of cereal. I only ate one plateful at dinner.

My mental health took a nosedive and I was readmitted to the psychiatric ward at the university. I had a routine blood test that all patients were given.

"Sandra," said a nurse, "You're highly dehydrated and have a deficiency of salt in your body. You need to drink four 8-ounce glasses of tomato juice a day."

"For how long?"

"At least three months or until you are better."

I substituted V-8 juice. Slowly, I restored the water content in my body. The salt helped me to rehydrate. My symptoms subsided. I was discharged.

That summer our family went on vacation to Hawaii with another family. We had a wonderful time. Things were looking up. I felt refreshed and content despite sunburn. Hope for the future motivated me to keep striving.

From Rehospitalization to the Senior Prom

September 1981 - July 1983

My family didn't think less of me despite my illness. They witnessed my repeated cycles of highs and lows. It's painful to see a loved one experience the types of things I experienced. My behavior was so erratic, my parents didn't know one day from the next how I would react. Ava was the most resilient of us all. At the dinner table, she made clever, funny remarks to break the tension. She felt it was her job to cheer people up. She rarely showed any pain or fear; instead she put on a happy face and helped us to laugh at ourselves and be a family.

Outside of the immediate family, few of my relatives knew I had a mental illness. My parents and sisters were my caregivers. They had little knowledge about mental illness initially, but saw the effects it had on me. No one gave them a crash course in psychiatry to explain about symptoms and medications. Instead, they learned ways to deal with me on a day-to-day basis. When I got upset, they'd comfort me. When I was hungry, they cooked meals. I was expected to do chores and keep my room clean. I did my homework diligently.

Our family appeared to be in harmony when guests came to the house. There were days when each of us dealt with our own crises. We lived and slept under the same roof but the communication was weak. I shared with my sisters, but they were facing their own dilemmas at that age.

My mother rose to the occasion as a working mom. She worked full-time but still had dinner on the table or made sure we took turns cooking. I disliked cooking dinner and wanted to find a way to get around it. I called my father at work one afternoon.

"Hey dad, I'm cooking a special dinner tonight. Make sure you're home on time for supper because I want it to be perfect."

"Sure, thanks." He sounded pleased.

I started to cook supper. I put every sauce I could find in the refrigerator and poured it onto the rice, vegetables, and beef strips I was cooking. I tested it to make sure it had too much seasoning. It was the worst dish one could imagine. Through this intentional trick, I hoped I would no longer be asked to cook.

My father arrived home with a smile on his face. He sat down to eat and I took the lid off his plate.

"What's this?" Doubtfully, he looked at the black sauce on the overcooked food.

"It's the special dinner I cooked for you dad. Eat up!"

After a short hesitation, he slowly picked up a fork and took a bite. He spit it out. The others picked at their food. My sister ran for the fridge to wash down the salty taste with milk. As I glanced around the table, no one looked very happy.

After that, to my satisfaction, I was no longer asked to cook dinner.

Gardening was another thing I disliked. It was a real effort for me to rake, prune, or tend the garden. Physically, I wasn't a strong person. I was also sensitive to sunlight because of my medication. I could easily become overheated or dehydrated. My mother would make a deal with me. If I spent an hour gardening, I could do whatever I wanted for the rest of the day.

At 4 P.M. on weekdays, when my mother got home from work, she turned off the stereo I listened to after school. When she was home, I couldn't play loud music. She was the type of mother who believed reading was more beneficial than watching television. She reinforced strong moral values and the importance of conscience. If my sisters or I did something wrong, we knew enough to feel guilty about it. My parents were strong disciplinarians and expected their three daughters to obey the rules of the house and go to church.

I was asked to pray before dinner but I refused. During my first psychotic break, I stopped going to church. My mother would try everything in her power to get me out of bed to go to church on Sunday mornings. Her faith in God gave her hope that I would recover.

But I had my doubts. I questioned why God let me suffer. Why did he allow schizophrenia to take over my life?

During hardship, some people lose faith while others find theirs. Because I believed God was punishing me, I chose to opt out of Sunday services. But later on, I did return to the church for a year. I sang in the choir. I loved to sing because it made me feel joy. I also participated in Friday night youth groups sponsored by the church. We went roller-skating and ice-skating. We enjoyed social functions, ate meals together, and developed friendships with each other.

I knew my parents clung to their beliefs which strengthened their resolve and hope for the future of their children.

I didn't have that sort of faith. I wondered if God wished the illness on me. I felt enormous guilt and shame. Years later, I still couldn't reconcile a benevolent God with the hardships I faced daily.

I wondered if I'd been born into a different family, if my life would have turned out better. Was my illness a result of my upbringing?

"Would you say I was neglected as a child?" I asked Dr. White. "If they'd given me more attention, maybe I wouldn't have felt so inferior and developed this illness."

"It's a common fallacy that bad parenting is to blame for mental illness. Even though you think your home life was difficult at times, that is not the reason you got ill," she replied. "Some people live in the best of homes and still may become ill. Your illness is caused by a chemical imbalance in the brain. Your family used to have poor communication but they are trying to make it better."

Once my family acknowledged my illness, they took care of my basic needs. In some ways, I felt emotionally neglected but I shut out others as much as they attempted to empathize with me. My life would have turned out very differently if my family abandoned me or sent me packing at eighteen. Despite the difficulty of living with a mentally ill person, they never rejected me. They did the best they could.

#

In sessions with Dr. White, conversations didn't always go well.

70

"You're not helping me. I'm wasting my time with you," I complained. "You aren't a good psychiatrist." I was frustrated I hadn't made enough progress.

"I can't cure you." Her next words surprised me. "I have something to say. I'm leaving for Thailand to study holistic medicine."

Immediately, I flipped from accusation to apology. "I'm sorry if I made you want to leave because of mean things I might have said."

I accept your apology but my reasons to leave are my own." She hugged me. "Dr. Franklin will see you now. Good luck."

After two years of therapy sessions with Dr. White, I left on a high note. I knew she was entering a time of new discovery and could potentially find other alternatives to patient care. It was also time for me to move on. We had outgrown each other.

I wrote her a letter years later. I found her address in the phone book. I wrote that she had been a major component in my recovery. She sent me a postcard that read, "It's people like you that make it all worthwhile."

#

In the fall of my final high school year, Penny was overseas, teaching English and traveling. I called her long distance when I was experiencing difficulty. "Please come back! I need you. I'm so crazed." I bawled on the phone.

She got on a plane and flew back to Vancouver. She was there for me and took time away from her life overseas to help and comfort me. Things got better for me but I knew she wished to return to Asia. It was a personal sacrifice for her to come back at that time. She really loved me.

71

I was admitted to the psychiatric ward at another hospital near my home. This time, I thought the other patients were actors and actresses from *Poldark*, a 1975 TV series. I believed their presence was part of the plot to confuse and destroy me. They were testing my limits.

My new psychiatrist, Dr. Franklin, gave me positive feedback but I was still not well.

"If it's all a farce, I'm not fit for anything except to return to hospital," I told him. I burst into tears and covered my face with my hands. I was filled with self-loathing. How could this happen to me?

At that point, I developed the full-blown delusion that I was a psychiatric experiment. In later years, I spoke with other people with mental illness, who believed at times they were an experiment too. It wasn't unique to me.

I decided the doctors were observing my behavior and symptoms to study the illness and find a cure. They had induced schizophrenia in me. By keeping me ill, they could continue their research. They hampered my ability to succeed in order to control my life and create enough stress to study my reactions.

On the other hand, if I was a psychiatric experiment and a cure was found I would receive the Nobel Prize. Because of my telepathic ability, they could also record my thoughts, which I communicated to Darren and others.

Most people would find my notion of being a test subject with ESP absurd, but in my mind I built a belief structure that was hard to break. It was escapism with a capital "E."

I asked myself, "Would such an experiment be ethical?" I remembered signing a waiver in the hospital and believed that in signing the document, I agreed to participate willingly. Perhaps my parents agreed to it because they believed I was a genius and my role in the experiment was my contribution to aid those less fortunate than me. Because of their cooperation, I imagined that my father, who was an architect, was rewarded with building contracts. I believed the doctors thought it was ethical because the outcome would be a cure.

I thought that Darren actively spied on me, was malicious, and ultimately caused me to become ill. In regards to Darren's criminal actions against me, which I believed were to undermine my cognitive abilities, and scare and fool me into thinking I was mentally ill, he would never be charged because he was a minor.

After he became an adult, any black marks on his record would be sealed and he was protected legally. He had extreme power over me. I had no defenses against him and yielded to him as if under hypnotic control. Still I could not separate the real Darren from the one created in my mind.

On the psychiatric ward, I met up with Jason again who had come on to me in the music room at the University Hospital psychiatric ward. He asked me to give him a massage. He said he'd pay me for it. I agreed. He told me to meet him in his room. On his bed, I straddled his body and began to massage his back. Soon he was on top of me, caressing me again. I said, "I don't want to do this."

He stopped right away. He grabbed a camera and began to take pictures of me. I tried to shield my face. He smiled, took the film out of the camera and exposed it to the light.

In my mind, I believed he was a drummer in a famous band. The real drummer had died of an overdose, but I believed Jason was indeed the same person, and had faked his death because he became mentally ill and didn't want the public to know. My fascination that he was a superstar made me vulnerable to his advances.

After three weeks, I was discharged and returned to school.

#

The following January, my mental health declined. I was admitted to a youth ward at the hospital. Every time I visited or slept on a ward, I smelled a disinfectant odor. It wasn't only in the sleeping quarters and washrooms, but the halls and stairways. The odor in hospitals is unlike any other. I'd want to wash the smell off me, but as long as I was there, it was in my nostrils all the time.

On the youth ward, I shared a room with another girl. I wasn't sure why she was there. She seemed normal enough. Another girl punched me in the shoulder every time she saw me. It wasn't long before I had a bruised arm.

We watched videos, went on group outings to the aquarium and parks, and ate together. During the mornings, I had an algebra tutor and worked on some assignments. I wrote a funny fairy tale about the others on the ward, which I read to them.

"That's really funny," said one girl.

"She got David's last name wrong," criticized another.

"Don't worry, it isn't going to be published," I countered. They laughed.

I also had a sketchbook, which I showed to my

roommate. She said, "You draw very well. Can you draw me?"

After a day or so, the word got around that I had artistic talent. I did portraits of some of the patients. One of the staff offered to draw me. She drew a very clever cartoon that brought out my features. Then she asked me to draw her. After it was finished she said, "The likeness is very good. I'm Scandinavian and you caught those characteristics very well."

I saw a psychiatrist on the ward. She was physically attractive and wore cream-colored hosiery. I thought she would have made a good living as a model if she ever quit her job as a psychiatrist. "You don't have a problem in your head. I think you can grow out of this."

"Then why am I on medication? Why can't I just recover naturally?"

"You're stuck in the past. Don't let it control you."

Later one of the nurses said to me, "You have the most potential of any of the patients on this ward. We've never had such a good group of kids at one time. You are a good influence."

One day, I was playing with a tape recorder alone in my room with the door closed. I decided to play a trick on the staff. I knew they checked on me every half hour or hour. I heard a knock on the door. "Are you okay in there?"

"Yep. Just recording some tapes."

"Good. Dinner's in an hour."

"Oh, I wouldn't want to miss that," I said facetiously.

I left the tape recorder playing music, put on my shoes, and snuck out the door and down the hall.

At the entrance to the unit, the nursing station was empty. Keeping low, I was able to escape out the door. It buzzed as I opened it. I was sure they'd be after me in a matter of seconds. My heart pounded as I took the stairs two at a time, looking for the closest exit. Afraid of being seen, I ran down to the basement level. A maze of corridors led to other parts of the hospital complex. I wanted to use an indirect route because they would soon be after me. I ran into a washroom and crouched on the toilet seat in one of the cubicles.

I heard a female voice call out to me. "Come out. Now."

I stayed still, fearing detection. Maybe she didn't really know I was there and was just testing. If she really wanted me, wouldn't she yank me out of there instead of waiting for me to come out?

I decided I'd waited long enough and walked out of the washroom. Immediately, I felt a hand around my wrist.

"Come with me."

She took me back to the ward, pushing me from behind to make me walk faster. When we got to the ward, she grabbed me by the wrist and ordered me back to my room.

One of the psychiatrists on the ward had a word with me in private. "Why are you here?"

"Because I need emotional attention," I replied.

"You have a serious illness. This isn't a game. The fact you attempted to escape is against the law."

"I don't believe that."

"After being admitted, you fall under the jurisdiction of this hospital which is under the mandate of the provincial government. Any attempt to escape will not be dealt with lightly. If you're out there, we can't protect you. The alternative is living on the streets, drugs, and prostitution."

"My parents will take me back." It seemed simple to me.

"You're dismissed."

I thought he was using scare tactics so I wouldn't leave again but perhaps his warnings were accurate. Where would I have gone if I had escaped? Would I become prey to others?

I heard about cases of young girls being hooked on drugs working for pimps. I didn't want to become a face on a missing persons poster. I sobered up and didn't try to escape again.

As punishment, I wasn't allowed to leave the premises for supervised outings for two days or discuss my escape attempt with any of the other patients. They took the tape recorder away. I decided I didn't care.

Paula, a girl with brunette hair, was admitted a month after me. She was also diagnosed with paranoid schizophrenia.

"Talk with Paula. You have similarities," advised one of the psychiatric nurses.

After talking to her, I didn't think we had things in common other than our diagnoses. The other patients didn't like her.

#

Months later, I ran into Paula at a bus stop. We exchanged phone numbers. She invited me to her place in Burnaby and I took the bus to visit her. She waved and smiled when she saw me approach the door. She lived in a two level condominium.

"Do you live with your mom and dad?" I asked.

"Only my mother. She works at the prison," she replied. "Would you like some lunch?" She made me macaroni and cheese. We went up to her room and she showed me her collection of pills. She must have been taking at least fifteen pills and vitamins a day.

"Do you remember when we met at the bus stop?" She curled up on a wicker chair, facing me. Her bare feet rested on the edge of her seat.

"Yeah." I noticed she only had one small window in the bedroom covered by a curtain. It felt stuffy. The light was dim.

"I was going to the West End to visit someone," she said.

"Oh, really?" I answered, unsure of the direction the conversation was headed.

"A man pays me for sex. I make a lot of money."

"How did you meet him? How old is he?" I was curious but not judgmental.

"It doesn't really matter. He asks me to do weird things sometimes."

"Like what?"

"Urinate on him," she said in a neutral voice.

"Yuck. Does he use a condom?"

"Usually. My mother told me if I'm going to have sex I have to take birth control pills."

"What about sexually transmitted diseases?"

"I'm not worried about that."

"Do you like him?" I asked. "If I had sex I'd want to

be in love with the person. Isn't that more meaningful?"

"There's nothing wrong with what I do."

"How can you say that?"

"If he wasn't paying me, he'd pay someone else. Why not me? I can buy things."

On the bus route home, I wondered about her. As long as she was willing to prostitute her body, nothing anyone said would change her behavior. I really didn't know the appropriate response. She called me the next day to thank me for coming.

"I feel bad about what you told me," I confessed.

"Why? I have nothing to hide." She seemed so candid. "I remember you said you were an artist."

"Yeah, I paint."

"Can you give me a painting?"

"I don't think so. I really want to market my paintings for sale."

"I'll show all my friends and hang it where people can see it. When can I come by to pick it up?"

"You don't even know if you like my art." I stalled.

"Of course I will. Please!!"

I had mixed feelings about this girl. I felt sorry for her so I decided to give her a painting.

Paula arrived on my doorstep an hour later. I passed her a painting of flower pods. She tugged it out of my hands, smiled and said goodbye. I didn't contact her after that.

I heard descriptions of past abuse or self-harm from others with mental illness. I found it difficult to not be shocked and to respond in a positive or helpful manner because I had no solutions to their problems. I found such conversations disturbing despite my own situation.

#

When I was discharged from the hospital, I got a phone call from an acquaintance named Greg. I had met him at camp and the youth group I attended. He was eight years older than me. He was of Scottish descent, blond and blue-eyed.

"Hi Sandra. Greg here. Would you like to go for a drink?"

"I don't drink. I'm underage."

"I meant lemonade," he said.

We met and took a walk. We ate ice cream in the park and went for lasagna at a local restaurant. He'd show up on my doorstep just to say hello. Soon we were dating regularly. I didn't talk much about my symptoms or illness. By that time, I had stabilized on my medication.

#

During my last year in high school, I took a reduced number of courses to cut down on my stress level. I opted for creative writing, sewing and art rather than English literature, biology or chemistry. I didn't take grade twelve social studies either.

My counselor assured me, "Even if you don't finish all your classes or miss some credits, you will still graduate."

"Even if I fail a final exam?"

"I've talked to the principal. You will graduate on merit if needed. We think you are bright enough to graduate even if you don't take all the requisite courses."

"Will I be able to continue to college or university?"

"That depends on you."

My date for the prom was Karl Guitterman. We didn't choose our dates. They were drawn randomly and assigned to us. I was relieved because I was guaranteed a date and wouldn't have to go alone.

I sewed a mauve satin dress with a low back to wear. Karl came to my house to take me to the graduation dinner at a hotel downtown. I was so nervous that my shoulders trembled and my heart beat rapidly. He pinned a corsage to my dress and escorted me to the car.

Dinner was shrimp cocktail, salad, chicken, roast potatoes, and cheesecake for dessert. I didn't say much over dinner. I was so nervous that my hand shook as I held my soupspoon. The valedictorian and class president gave speeches. We toasted to our friends and futures.

After dinner, my nervousness became fear.

"Karl, can you take me home?"

"Why? The party's just started," he answered.

"No, I need to go home now." I stood up and put on my coat.

"It's early. Please stay."

I don't know the reason for my apprehension. I imagined a fight would break out or something worse. He drove me home in silence and kissed me good night. I thanked him and went inside. He called me fifteen minutes later.

"Can I come and get you? There's lots of entertainment happening here. I don't want you to miss out." I could hear music and laughter in the background.

"No, I'm going to bed." I said good-bye and hung up the phone.

That was my graduation. No loud parties, drinking

or dancing that night. I spent the rest of the evening lying in bed, with the radio on, staring at the light hanging from the ceiling. In a catatonic state, I was oblivious to the outside world. It may seem odd that I didn't want to celebrate with my fellow students. Instead I was drawn into my own world.

Memories of the past five years seemed to fade in intensity. I missed segments of my life, now forgotten. I was leaving my youth and entering a new phase.

Fighting Through School on Prescribed Drugs

August 1983 - June 1989

After high school, I wanted to attend a fine arts program at a community college. I envisioned becoming an artist as a career. To qualify, each candidate had to appear for an interview with a portfolio and submit a high school transcript.

"Hello, I'm Tom Hunter, sculpture instructor." He shook my hand with a firm grip. He had long hair in a ponytail and a full beard. "Let's get to it. What's in your portfolio?"

I pulled out a sketchpad of drawings and paintings that I completed in grade twelve. He pointed at one drawing. "This is a self-portrait."

I nodded.

He held up a photo of a Norman Rockwell painting I did and thumbed through my drawings. "Not bad. I see you've also included some nudes."

"I took a life drawing class."

"Very sensitive technique. I quite like it. Okay, that's all I need to see."

He shook my hand. Two weeks later I was notified that I had been accepted. Delighted, I shared the news with my family.

"Of course, you'd get in. I didn't doubt it," said my father.

"I can't even draw a straight line," said Ava.

"Use a ruler," interjected my dad. We laughed.

My mother called us to the dinner table. We talked and shared a scrumptious roast beef dinner. It was a good time for us.

#

I didn't share with anyone at college that I had a mental illness. I kept my big secret from my teachers and fellow students. Instead, I engrossed myself in learning various techniques in sculpture, ceramics, drawing, design, and painting.

Dr. Franklin was open to lowering my medication so I had enough energy to attend college. It was a balancing act to find a dosage, which controlled my symptoms enough but still allowed for creativity. I took trifluoperazine, trazodone, and lithium. The medication reduced emotional upheaval and paranoia but also my self-expression. The negative side effects included stiffness of joints, anxiety, tremors, sore throat, slurred speech, blurred vision, and mannerisms. I bounced when I walked and held my hands in a cupped position at all times. Even if I didn't tell anyone my big secret, I think they still knew I was on some type of medication.

Artists are a unique bunch. The stereotypical artist leads a bohemian lifestyle, may be alcoholic, and have angst or depression. The public is willing to accept the idea of the mad artist whose inner demons allow creativity to flow. So to be a painter was a logical choice for me. I fit in with the art crowd. We'd come up from the basement where the studios were located and go for coffee in the cafeteria with paint and plaster on our clothes. A lot of the art students smoked, but I didn't. We appeared different from the academic students with our dyed hair and stained clothes.

I enjoyed the studio classes as well as art history and English classes. I thrived on creative energy and socialized with other students. I learned about composition, balance, color mixing, and perspective in design class. I attempted the pottery wheel and managed to make several bowls and pots with lids. In sculpture class, I made a plaster mold and cast of my right hand, four times actual size. I received an honorable mention in printmaking to great applause from my fellow students. Mostly, I enjoyed acrylic painting.

My instructor said, "You are natural at printmaking. The technique is an extension of your creative process. It's as easy as drawing for you."

"I prefer painting," I answered.

"You can always paint for your own enjoyment. It's a matter of finding your best medium."

#

During summer break, I went on an art history tour in Europe with one of the art history professors. Twelve of us signed up. My parents paid my way. For three weeks, we traveled from London, to Amsterdam, Germany, Switzerland, Italy, and France. The trip was an amazing experience. I saw architecture and art that I had only seen on slides or in books. It all took my breath away.

We took walking tours through some of the cities. Highlights were the canals in Amsterdam; the Swiss Alps; the Sistine Chapel and St. Peter's Cathedral in Rome; St. Mark's Square and the canals in Venice; the Jeu de Paume and the Centre Pompidou in Paris; and the National Gallery and the Changing of the Guard in London.

One morning on a tour bus in southern France, our

leader, the art history professor, opened a bottle of champagne and I took a glass, even though my pill bottles warned not to mix alcohol with my medication. I felt giddy and warm. I had a very low tolerance for alcohol. I decided to stop taking my medication.

By the time we got to Paris, I passed on visiting the Louvre because I wanted to just goof off and shop at the tourist stalls.

In Paris, I drank half a beer, which was enough for me to lose my equilibrium. I staggered until the effects wore off.

When I got on the plane at Heathrow Airport in London to return home, I had developed a bad cough. I coughed continuously all the way home.

Arriving in Vancouver, I had jet lag and bronchitis as well as the effects of stopping my medication. Greg and my family met me at the airport.

The next night, my parents asked me into their bedroom for a talk.

"We are concerned because we don't think Greg's right for you," my mother said. "You need to date a Christian."

I rolled my eyes. "Who says I'm a Christian? Who would you like me to date?" I felt the conversation was absurd. I hadn't been to church for a long while. I was so distant from religion in general.

There's a passage someone wrote about footprints in the sand. A man looks back and sees only one set of footprints behind him. The man says, "Lord, why did you forsake me and allow me to suffer alone?"

The Lord answers, "I never forsook you. There is

only one set of footprints because I carried you."

I think about that story and I get so inflamed. I believed God never carried me. I rejected living within the confines of scripture. I wanted to make my own decisions.

As the conversation with my parents continued, I became angry and refused to break up with Greg. I was mad they judged him badly because he wasn't a Christian. Greg wasn't a hypocrite, a criminal or a bad person. He'd done more for me than any of my friends. If they wanted me to end that relationship, my life might have taken a different direction and not necessarily a good one. Greg was in my life for a reason.

I called Greg and met him the next day. "I don't care what they say. Suddenly, they have to fix my life that doesn't need fixing."

"I'm good for you. I know I'm a good person," said Greg grimly.

I decided not to heed my parents' objection. Greg and I continued our relationship. I moved temporarily to my grandparents' condominium, which was close to the college. I had trouble getting up in the morning so the move made sense because I could walk rather than travel by bus. I saw Greg often, walking to meet him halfway between his home and the condo. My parents had no control over my leisure time.

#

My Gung Gung suffered a series of strokes. When he was living at home with some impairment from his first stroke, he had been warned not to drive. But, he wanted to take his grandchildren to lunch at a family restaurant. He told us to put our shoes on and get in the car. He got in and put the car in reverse. I smiled at my sisters about this unusual adventure. He pulled out of the garage with no problem and set off down the street to the restaurant several miles away. I noticed he stayed well to the right to let other cars pass. He drove slowly so the car wouldn't swerve.

We enjoyed hamburgers and fries. Grandfather laughed and ate a little bit. He drove us home, again staying well to the right of the road. He parked and smiled.

"Grandma will never know," he said. It was our secret.

Later after another stroke, he was admitted to a rehabilitation facility. He couldn't talk but still had some cognitive ability. I went to see him several times. He seemed very frustrated that he couldn't talk. Arrangements were made to move him to long-term care.

One morning, my dad called the condo and said, "Stay with Po Po. We're coming over. Stay put."

I knew something was wrong. Ten minutes later, my dad and mom arrived at the door. "He passed away an hour ago," mom said. "He refused to eat. He knew the end was coming."

Po Po wailed. I'd never seen anyone grieve like that before. I didn't know how to respond. My own problems seemed so insignificant when I realized the loss of my grandfather and witnessed the grief of my grandmother and other relatives.

Preparations were made for the funeral. At the last minute, I decided I couldn't go because I was too disoriented to cope with the funeral. My mother's friend took me out instead. She treated me to lunch and we went to the mall. I denied anything was wrong when she asked me how I felt.

The next week I was walking down the street and I thought I saw my grandfather drive out of a garage and down the street. The driver wasn't really him but I wished he were still alive.

#

I found myself through art classes. I learned there are many correct ways to draw and paint. I found satisfaction in the creative process.

I painted in acrylics. In the beginning, I painted from my imagination, influenced by Picasso and Matisse. Painting was a healthy way to express my emotions. It cleared my mind of obsessive thoughts.

Art can be healing. To pull out a pen or pencil and sketch in the park is good therapy. The artists I've met do it because they enjoy it. To sell a painting makes me extremely happy but to receive compliments is rewarding too. I remember a time when I couldn't sell anything.

Someone told me that fantasies or delusions might in fact elevate my senses and aid me in increasing my creativity. I think perhaps he was right. My imagination and mood come through in my art. I may see things differently than others but perhaps that's a gift - not a bad thing.

I went through periods where I couldn't paint at all because of side effects of medication. It affected my fine motor skills and my ability to be spontaneous and free which are necessary qualities for an artist. At times, I had limited awareness of things around me and my responses were slowed because of the medication.

Making art was a journey. For me, the process reflected an inner struggle. I had no fixed plan when I start other than a thumbnail sketch or a photograph. I let the art evolve on its own. Some of my best work was the result of exploration with subject matter, color, texture and form.

When I put down one color of paint, then the next and blended them together, I created a visual dialogue without words or explanation. When I saw the finished product, I was proud of my efforts.

Some days, I painted at home with an old easel of my father's. After painting, I'd leave my paper palette to dry and toss out later. Once, I went downstairs to check on my painting and noticed paw prints of paint leading from my palette, over the table, and across the parquet floor. I scrubbed the prints off the floor as best as I could, but I always remembered how funny it was that our cat climbed up, walked in my paints and marked a trail behind her.

\#

I graduated from the Fine Arts program, moved back home, and transferred to university to study art history. My hard work for two years at college was rewarded with a government scholarship. The painting instructor encouraged me to apply to a fine art college but I wanted to try university as an academic student. After two years of intense art classes, I felt my creativity was temporarily depleted.

During this time, I had my first art show at a library in Port Coquitlam. I exhibited over twenty paintings and received two reviews in local newspapers. I was pleased to read the headline, "Shocking art helps her" and the article about teenage angst fueling my body of work. The paintings were psychological portraits based on my imagination.

The librarian, who was in charge of exhibitions, described my early paintings as an expression of the yin and yang in Chinese philosophy in a news release. The yin is dark, feminine, passive and corresponds to the night. The yang is light, masculine, active and relates to the day. So these contrasts create a tension; one cannot exist without the other. Likewise, in my painting, these two opposing forces came together in a dynamic way.

Greg introduced me to illustrative art as well as comic book artists like Gene Colan, Bill Sienkiewicz and Michael Kaluta. My paintings displayed comic book influences with their hard lines and bright colors. I received many wonderful comments in my guest book.

#

In the fall, I signed up for a full course load at the University of British Columbia (UBC). I had to make up some classes but I was eligible for third year art history courses. Greg had a degree already, but decided to apply for a one-year art history diploma.

We both enrolled in North American Architecture, History of Film, and Art Theory and Criticism. Without his help to study and search the libraries, I doubt I could have made it through. We'd eat lunch in the library. I'd take a nap everyday because I was so tired from the medication.

In the evenings, I'd study with Greg to memorize facts and images of art and architecture. I couldn't retain things very well and couldn't keep up taking notes in class. I'd forget to bring paper to class to record the information. Frustrated, I gave up taking notes and just listened to the

91

lectures.

Over a six-year period, I fought my way through college and university. I use the word "fought" because it was a battle everyday. The other students weren't on trifluoperazine, trazodone or lithium. They weren't dealing with mania, depression or delusions like me, or so I assumed. Between the medication and the illness, my ability to learn and concentrate was reduced compared to the alertness, intelligence and capabilities of the other students who advanced steadily. At that time, there were no counseling offices available to aid students with mental health problems like now.

I got through the school year but was upset with some of my grades. I wanted to get the same high grades that I received in high school, but that wasn't the case at university. My favorite course was Art Theory and Criticism. In the first term, I had A's on an in-class exam and a paper, but I received a passing grade at the end of the second term. I called the professor to ask why I had received such a low grade in comparison to my marks in the first term. She said she was very disappointed with my final paper. I thought about arguing the grade but was afraid I might lose the grade I did get. At least I passed, I thought. At the time I didn't plan on continuing on to postgraduate work, so I let it go.

During the summer, I took two geography courses to make up credits to be admitted to fourth year. When I reached the fourth year level, Greg had finished his diploma. I registered and bought books for the next set of courses. In September, I started to think members of my class were rock stars. I became afraid I would fail and cried in the women's washroom between classes. Fearing a relapse, I panicked and withdrew from all my courses.

Unsure of my direction, I floundered, wondering if I should look for work or try to re-enroll with a reduced course load. I decided to apply at an art college. I went for an interview and signed up for relief printmaking and drawing courses in January.

Unable to generate new ideas, I rehashed old drawings from my sketchbook into linocuts. Drawing class was uninspiring. I decided this particular art school wasn't the right choice for me.

#

During the summer, I wanted to find work to help pay for expenses. My parents were generous enough to pay my tuition, but I thought work experience would be good for me. I applied at several places and got an interview at a dress shop.

"Have you worked before?" The manager of the store looked at me over her bifocal glasses. She dressed well and wore thick make-up. I wondered how long she took to put on her make-up in the morning. I could smell her perfume.

"Yes, at an architect's office and a fabric store."

"So you have experience as a receptionist?"

"It was a long time ago." I had been a teenager at the time, working at my father's firm for one summer. I tapped my fingers on my knee restlessly.

"What did you learn from working in an office?"

"How to act professional and answer the phone."

"Why do you want this job?"

"Because I think it's a good learning experience and I

like people and working in sales." I gave her a big smile.

"And?"

I hesitated. What did she want me to say?

"You want to get paid, right?"

"Oh, yes!"

I was hired for the summer. I got along with the other salesgirls. They were friendly. I didn't tell them my big secret either. Sunday shift was the worst. There were hardly any customers in the lingerie department on Sundays. I felt so tired and hungry. I felt like napping. I tried to eat more before my shift, but I still yawned continually and my eyes would tear.

We didn't work on commission but the clerks with the highest three sales records got a bonus. I received a bonus twice in the first month I worked there. I became bored quickly and decided I'd rather goof off the rest of the summer.

"I have a health problem and I need to quit," I said to the manager.

"What kind of health problem?" she asked.

"That's confidential information."

I left at the beginning of August and spent time with Greg instead.

#

I re-enrolled at university the next fall, taking a reduced course load. Again, I was disappointed with my grades. Later on, I discovered people didn't really care about the percentage I got in a particular class. It didn't really matter in the long run as long as I made it through.

I still had daily challenges because of recurring symptoms and side effects from the medications. I would have bouts of depression lasting weeks. I cried so hard that I thought I damaged my brain cells. I still had delusions of writing songs on the radio or having ESP. One would think after awhile I should have been able to differentiate between symptom and reality but every time psychosis was triggered, I'd relapse into mental confusion, delusion and emotional upheaval.

My psychotic symptoms seemed arbitrary to others but not to me. Chains of fictitious events altered my sense of objectivity. I didn't live in a common reality, rather a seductive world where I was all knowing.

Because my delusions were so fantastic, I lived with my feet off the ground. As I stated before, psychosis was like a bad habit that gave me an initial buzz or feeling of invulnerability. In my head, I was a supreme being unequaled by anyone else. When I reached the climax of an episode, the house of cards I built with my mind would fall apart and I would plummet into deep depression. After exhausting my excess energy, I would calm down and insight would return. Then the cycle would repeat itself.

I was responsible enough to know I needed medication and I took it regularly. The older anti-psychotic medications like trifluoperazine and haloperidol may cause tardive dyskinesia, which consists of involuntary movements or tics like grimacing, puckering of the lips, rapid eye blinking or spasms of the arms or legs. Tardive dyskinesia is permanent. It continues even if the anti-psychotics are stopped.

My muscle rigidity and exaggerated gait were pronounced. I would constantly move my limbs because of restlessness caused by the medication.

I took Artane, which lessened the side effects of trifluoperazine but also had its own side effects.

Medication was a trade-off. In order to reduce my schizophrenic symptoms I had to take the medications, but they affected my academic performance and my ability to work. It was a catch-22.

While I was at university, Dr. Franklin adjusted my medication so I could get by. I'd go into his office and say I can't function well in the morning because I'm too sedated. He would drop my trifluoperazine by five milligrams. Three weeks later, I'd complain about the delusions returning, and he'd bump my dosage back up. It was a challenge to get up early to go to class and last until lunch. I'd wake up late and not eat a proper breakfast.

One day on the bus, I got dizzy and fainted. Other times in class I'd nod off. My mother lent me her car to drive to university. If I drove, I could leave later and concentrate on the road to keep me alert.

#

It took me longer than most students to finish university because I could only handle a few courses at a time. My last year included a course in Canadian Art. I liked Canadian Art class because it seemed more relevant to my own painting. I wanted to learn the history and trends in contemporary Canadian art. Where was mainstream art headed in the future? Unfortunately, I didn't find an answer to that question in the context of the course. We spent only a class or two on art in British Columbia.

Jack Shadbolt, one of my favorite B.C. artists, came to speak to the class. I was very pleased to see him in person. He had a good sense of humor and talked to us plainly. Later on, I wrote him two letters and he responded in handwritten letters. He died at age 89, leaving behind a legacy of art. I still consider him one of the major influences in my painting.

Again, I had difficulty taking notes in class and writing exams. I had few interfering thoughts, but the side effects of the medications caused me problems. I wanted to go off my medication, but Dr. Franklin advised against it.

"Sandra, do you feel it's the right dosage?"

"I'm tired, but what else is new," I said. I found it was a struggle to get up in the morning and hard to get to sleep at night. I had nightmares of being trapped, unable to move or talk. I had difficulty waking up because of sedation. "I think I can get by for the next few weeks. If, after that, I'm still having problems I'll let you know."

Dr. Franklin trusted me to be responsible that if I did have a downturn I would contact him. I trusted that he was looking out for me.

Throughout my schooling, despite my efforts, I remained stymied because of my mental confusion and medication, which dulled my ability to receive information. I was underdeveloped in some areas. I felt insecure. I had difficulty conversing with other students and especially the professors.

With some luck, I made it through my final year of university. My family was proud of me. The day of the graduation ceremony was a very extraordinary day not only for me but also for my mother. She graduated with a Master's degree in English Education the same day that I received a Bachelor of Arts in Art History. My mother participated in the morning ceremony and I was in the afternoon ceremony.

It was one of the happiest days of my life.

#

A family friend visited from Toronto. Sharon was a medical doctor, a musician and also a photographer. Because I knew she had creative talent, I showed her some of my art.

"You should be in a fine arts college," she said.

"I tried the art college here, but it wasn't the right place for me."

"You should study art in New York."

"I can't." I suddenly felt anxious.

"Why not?"

I blurted out, "Because I'm schizophrenic."

"That's no problem. You can still go to New York."

Alarm bells went off in my mind and my pulse quickened. How could I manage to live in a foreign city without the support of my family? How could I navigate finding a psychiatrist or getting prescriptions in New York? There was no way I could pay for tuition, supplies, books, a place to live, food, and psychiatric care. Certainly, Sharon as a medical doctor, must have known her suggestion was unrealistic and quite beyond my capabilities.

"I can't leave Vancouver. What if I get sick?"

"They have medications now that can eliminate your symptoms."

News to me, I thought. My medications didn't eliminate my symptoms. I shook my head. I felt it was so obvious that I was too weak and afraid to even consider a move to another city. A huge barrier came up.

She must have noticed my discomfort. "What if I take your picture?" The corners of her eyes crinkled when she smiled. "Come on. Let's check the light outside."

We went out onto the back deck. She squinted at the bright sun. "In an hour the light will be just right." Sure enough an hour later, the sunlight wasn't as strong but it was still daylight. She set up her camera and took four pictures of me with my paintings. I laughed as I took various poses and she snapped the photos.

A month after she returned to Toronto, I received four photographs in the mail. They were 8 by 10 inches and captured the true colors of my paintings. I was very pleased and mailed her a letter to thank her. Even though she was a doctor, she didn't understand the limitations I had because of my illness. On the other hand, she felt my art was good enough for art colleges in New York. She believed my illness shouldn't negatively impact my dream to be an artist.

#

My family was invited to a wedding and banquet dinner. I knew both the bride and groom who were about my age and wished the best for them. Many of my acquaintances and cousins married during the time I graduated and started working.

The banquet dinner was held at a hotel downtown. I sat next to a commerce professor, Anthony, I had known for a number of years.

"How's the art sales coming along?" he asked me.

"Oh, what art sales exactly?" I took a sip of water from a glass.

"You must be selling paintings. You're an artist."

99

"Yes, but I'm a starving artist."

"When you go to Hong Kong-"

"I'm not going to Hong Kong," I interjected.

"In Hong Kong, you can sell art. People will go for it."

"How do you know that?"

"Because everything sells in Hong Kong."

"By the time you factor in freight charges, travel, and accommodation, what's left?"

"Get an agent."

"So without knowing any Cantonese or Mandarin, I'm supposed to hop over to Hong Kong, make some contacts, get an agent, and deliver the work. So how do I stop them from taking all the revenue and spending it on dim sum?" I drummed my fingers on the table for effect.

"You have a contract."

"I don't think I'm ready for Hong Kong," I said. Soon the waiters served the first course and the conversation ended. It seemed so simple to him to suggest ways for me to market my work, but because of something I lacked, I didn't have the vision of selling my work overseas.

#

Another fellow that I knew was climbing the corporate ladder. He worked for a coffee company. I spoke to him one Sunday afternoon after a church service. It was a rare occasion when my mother actually got me to attend church. Coincidentally, we were both at the coffeemaker before the adult group convened for a discussion after the sermon.

"Hey, Sandra," he said to me. "How would you like

to submit a proposal for a mural for the interior of our building?"

"What kind of mural? Something to do with coffee, I suppose."

"Something that says 'corporate.' " He stirred his coffee.

"I don't paint abstract art."

"It doesn't have to be abstract. It can be anything you want."

"No nudity right?" I jested.

"I'm asking you on behalf of the company."

I said, "Sure, no problem." I walked away, cup in hand.

I put the conversation out of my head. Certainly, there was no way I could do a large mural that was good enough for a corporation. I wasn't a professional mural painter.

I didn't see him for a while, but he left a message on the phone that the deadline was coming up. The day of the deadline, he called me again.

"Sandra, it's five minutes before our meeting. I told the others that I was expecting a proposal. If you have something, please fax it to me now."

I was shocked. I couldn't believe he actually took his proposal seriously because I hadn't. Someone was knocking at the door and I missed it. If I had been open to at least attempting to check out the building and come up with preliminary sketches and an idea, I could have had the opportunity and experience of doing a major work for a corporation that could pay. Instead, I missed another chance to further myself. If I didn't take my art seriously, no one else would.

I visited the local drugstore to make some color photocopies of my art. I asked the pharmacist for the amount I was to pay. He glanced at the photocopies in my hand.

"Let me see," he said. He took the pictures from my hand. "You did these?"

I nodded.

"You have the originals?"

"Most of them." I had sold a few by then.

"You need to make prints. Always keep your originals. Do you have more of these?"

"I have a portfolio of lots of paintings."

"Bring it in. I want to see more."

Thinking he was pretty demanding, but curious to know his assessment of my work, I brought in my portfolio the next day. After he served the other customers, I passed my leather portfolio to him over the counter.

He studied the photos of my work. "Good. But I still say prints are the way to sell your work. If you sell an original, it's gone forever. But if you make copies, you can sell them like water."

"Like water?" I grinned.

"Haven't you heard of Giclee prints? It's a way of reproducing paintings on canvas."

I nodded. "How do I choose which paintings are the ones that I should reproduce?"

"The artist always knows which is her best work." He handed back the portfolio. "I've got work to do."

After that, whenever I saw him at the drugstore, he'd

102

ask about my progress in painting. I was amused that this pharmacist had such a strong interest in my career and his own expert advice on how to make money out of my art. But still, he was another example of someone who thought more of my art than I did at that time.

People came in and out of my life. Some carried messages that I ignored. I was blind to the opportunities that were possible. Instead, without the tools and knowledge to market my work, I stayed within the confines of my perception that my art wasn't good enough to sell. Maybe it wasn't so much my art wasn't ready for the world, but that I wasn't ready to share it.

The Challenge of Working

July 1989 - February 1994

My mother talked about living in the real world. She believed with hard work, one could achieve a life of independence. Once one graduated, she expected one should look for a job.

A Bachelor's degree in Art History doesn't amount to much in the world of employment in my experience. I could have chosen to work in a gallery but most commercial galleries will not accept green graduates from university unless they had experience or knowledge about contemporary art and references to back that up.

Some of the others in my classes went on to the Master's degree program, which would qualify them to teach. I wasn't interested in following that direction.

As most of my work experience was retail, I applied to work in sales at a dress shop on Fourth Avenue. I went for an interview.

"Have you worked on commission before?" The manager was quick to size me up.

I shook my head.

"We have a part-time and a full-time position available. If you could choose, which would be your choice?"

"Part-time."

"Why do you only want to work part-time? Wouldn't you earn more working full-time?"

"I need time for myself."

She raised an eyebrow. "Why?"

"To see people."

"Oh, you have a boyfriend?" I thought she was pretty presumptuous. "What does he do?" she inquired.

I felt rather uncomfortable. "He's a gardener."

"Oh, I'm looking for a gardener. I need someone to mow my lawn. It's on an incline and hard to cut. Would he be able to cut my lawn?"

I soon realized this wasn't the employer I wanted and applied elsewhere. I spoke to the manager of a boutique on Granville Street. They carried funky clothes at reasonable prices.

"Hello, I've just graduated from university. I saw your sign in the window and would like to apply for a sales position. I really like the clothes you sell. I'd love to work here."

She looked at my résumé. "Wait a moment please." She disappeared into the backroom of the store. After a few minutes, she came back out. "I checked with my supervisor. We don't usually do this, but since you're here already, how about an interview?"

I nodded and smiled and we went into the backroom. I gave her the best impression I could. She gave me the name of her supervisor for a second interview the next day.

I went for my second interview with the supervisor. I didn't know the owner was in the other room listening.

As we talked, I soon realized the company was a good match for me. I was hired as a sales clerk at the Granville store.

The assistant manager at the Granville store quit around the time I started work. Another sales clerk had been hired days after me. The manager took me aside.

"The assistant manager position has opened up. I could ask the other sales clerk if she wants the position, but because you were hired before her, we may offer it to you first."

"Oh, definitely, I'd like to be promoted." I'd been there three weeks.

"We have to make a decision. The job isn't yours yet," she said.

After the store closed that day, the supervisor dropped by to talk privately with the manager in the backroom. I knew that when the store closed, we had to cash out. So I entered the password and began the process of cashing out. The computer led me through the process. I counted the float and took out the money and checks to be deposited at the bank. I kept counting the cash, worried that the amount was three cents short.

The supervisor came out of the backroom.

"Is this right?" I asked her.

She looked at the computer printout and nodded.

"I'm afraid we're three cents out," I said. "I couldn't make it balance correctly."

"You're worried about three cents?" She was amused. "Did the manager teach you to cash out?"

"No, I just watched her do it."

After that, they were confident I could handle the assistant manager position and I received a promotion and a small raise. I didn't tell them I had figured out the password without being told.

After that, I worked Sundays to Thursdays. It was physical work to merchandise, receive stock, and steam the clothes. I spent part of my paycheck on clothes from the store. I made signs to feature sale items.

One day, I lost my keys including my car key, house key and the one for the store. My manager was afraid that someone would find the keys and rob the store. She called the owner to request a change in the locks. The day the locksmith was to arrive, the manager was taking out the trash. She heard a clinking sound coming from the garbage bag. She opened it up and found my keys. Immediately, she told me. I figured the keys had fallen into the wastebasket accidentally from a shelf below the counter where I had put them. She called the owner to cancel the locksmith's appointment. I watched my keys carefully after that.

Regular customers who lived or worked in the area would come in to buy or browse. One old lady came in and I greeted her. She looked closely at my face.

"You're a Christian. I see the presence of God in you," she said.

I grinned at her. "I think you see God in yourself."

"Praise the Lord." She clasped her hands and left.

I heard other people also say I had a glow about me. It was quite the compliment.

One lady came in often near closing time, hoping to get a good deal by making a nuisance. We gave her free shoulder pads but no discounts.

One woman got angry because she wanted to return an item and the store was closed.

"We're closed. Come back tomorrow." I said from behind the locked glass door.

"I'm not in town tomorrow. I live in White Rock. Look I just want to return this item." Outside, she waved a pair of shorts in her hand.

"We aren't allowed to open the door after closing. We're cashing out."

"I want my money back."

I looked at the manager. She looked back at me. "How do I deal with her? Can we let her in?" I didn't know the proper way to handle the angry customer.

The manager shrugged. "We have rules. The store's closed." After a while, the woman gave up and left. I guess we lost a customer that day.

After eight months of working full-time, I was exhausted. I needed a holiday or some time off but didn't ask for it. My family planned a trip to Cancun, Mexico. I was afraid to ask for time off to go with them. Vacation time was scheduled by order of seniority. I could have asked for time off without pay, but I didn't. The week my family was away enjoying the hot sun, staying at a resort, I worked six days in a row because my manager was on a buying trip with the owner in Montreal. By the next week, I couldn't cope. Drained, I called in sick.

"Will you be back this afternoon?" asked my manager.

"I need a week off," I said.

"Why a whole week?"

"I can't work. I'm not well."

"Okay, but it will go on your record." She said goodbye.

I hung up the phone.

She called me the next day. "Someone canceled their shift. Can you come in this afternoon?"

Not quite awake at nine in the morning, I agreed. An

hour later, fully awake, I called back to say I couldn't work. That didn't sit well with the manager. I told her I had to speak with her. She met me at the diner next to the store.

I walked in and sat down. She lit up a cigarette. "What are you going to tell me? We aren't happy, kid."

I felt slighted. She was younger than me. "I have to quit. I have paranoid schizophrenia and I can't work because of stress and fatigue."

"That's funny. I never met someone like you before. Did this craziness happen recently?"

"I've been ill since grade nine."

"So you're telling me suddenly you can't work because you're schizoid?" She puffed on her cigarette.

"I take medication to stabilize."

"Hmm, I've heard a lot of excuses, but I guess you're not making this one up. Quit if you want."

"I'm putting in my resignation. Do you want me to work a couple of weeks so you have time to find a replacement?"

"We certainly don't want you working at the store if you're so ill. It's better if you don't come back. I think a clean break is best." She took a drag on her cigarette and put it out.

The manager's derisive comments cut into me. I knew I deserved respect but didn't pursue it. I felt discriminated because of her attitude.

Later, I realized the real world that my mother talked about was only an abstract concept. In life, people have different roles and situations. Their goals and lifestyles varied. Did I really want to live in the real world rather than my own fictional version? It was safer to believe others were in charge of my life in secret rather than face the reality that my life depended on my own initiative to get ahead without a safety net. My family was behind me but my future depended on my ability to survive, make smart choices, and build a life for myself.

#

I taught several after school art classes to elementary students in Burnaby. It was a paid position to work a two-hour shift one day a week. I learned that when children get out of school at the end of the day, all they want to do is play and have a break. Some of the classes went very well, others were out of control. I don't know if it was my fault that I couldn't keep the class focused. Kids will be kids. The art classes were meant to be a leisure activity. Nothing they did in an art class was wrong as long as they didn't throw paint or glue around. The kids enjoyed making pop-up cards with the fluorescent paper I supplied.

Teaching kite making was a little more difficult. I found simple kite instructions and did a couple of samples as a trial run. The best part about kite making class that was once we finished the kites; we went outside and tested them. Normally, once the kite is in the air, one doesn't have to move much other than to adjust the tension on the line, but my students liked to run around to keep the kites in the air.

I got a call from the supervisor of the clothing store on Granville Street where I had worked before.

"Hello Sandra, I heard you were looking for work. If you are interested you can reapply."

"I don't want to be assistant manager. It was too stressful."

110

"Would you like to meet the new manager and me to talk about it?"

"Sure. Where and when?"

I noted the time and place and told my sister Ava the news. She seemed doubtful. "How did they know you were looking for work?"

"I mentioned it to one of the staff," I responded.

"Are you sure you want to go back there?"

"What else am I qualified to do? I only know retail," I said. "The previous manager is gone. Maybe if I work part-time I won't burn out."

"It's your decision, but make sure it's the right one," she advised.

I arrived at the coffee shop, eagerly met by the supervisor and new manager. After five minutes, I offered to return to work for them.

So I returned to work as a part-time salesperson, but I became bored quickly. To say "May I get you a fitting room? I'm here if you need another size," or "That's washable silk. Just hang it to dry" over and over again was part of the job. I hinted to the manager that I wasn't happy in my demoted position.

A new sales clerk was hired.

"Has anyone showed you how to use the cash register?" I asked her on her second day.

She shook her head.

"How can you work here without knowing how to use it? I'll show you. Use my employee code until you get your own."

Taking initiative to train her was the wrong thing to do. The reason the manager didn't show her how to use the register was because she wasn't ready. She quit soon after for personal reasons.

The new assistant manager looked like she was sixteen. I helped her out when she seemed uncertain. She quit too. I thought I could easily step into the job since I did some of her work for her anyway. "Do you need a new assistant manager?" I asked the manager.

"Why do you ask?"

"Well, I could do it for you in the interim until you find someone," I offered.

"Didn't you say last week you weren't happy here and now you want to be assistant manager?"

"Did I say that? I'm trying to help you out."

"You hinted you were looking for another job. We don't know if you're going to be here next week or the week after."

I realized I no longer wanted the job and the manager wasn't thrilled about me either. It was time to move on.

#

I asked my father if I could work in his architectural firm as a secretary. He didn't interview me or ask for a résumé. He only said, "Be here tomorrow at nine." He usually left for work at 7:30 or 8 A.M. I was unable to rise early because of my sedating medication. Instead, I arrived ten minutes late after nine.

The first day, I sat at the reception desk. The phone rang about four times an hour. My father left to go to city hall. My eyes started to tear and my head nodded as I tried to stay awake. My medication dosage had been increased and it fogged my mind. By 2 P.M., he hadn't returned. I didn't have a key to lock up the office so I couldn't leave for lunch. I waited. Finally he showed up in the afternoon.

"Can I have a key to the office?" My voice slurred from the medication.

"There's one in the drawer."

"It was there the whole time? I'm so hungry and tired that I want to go home."

"Have some coffee."

My father and I would lunch together at a restaurant adjacent to the office building. Often we'd join an accountant who ate there regularly. We had great conversations about economics, politics, architecture, and current events. They were good friends and had business dealings together.

Work was slow at the office. There wasn't much for me to do except open the mail, balance the general ledger, and pay bills.

The phone rang off the hook between noon and one. My father would always take the calls. I desperately wanted to go for lunch, which was the highlight of my workday. "We can't go for lunch on time, if you keep taking calls," I complained.

"In that case, take the phone off the hook," he suggested.

"Why don't we get an answering machine?"

"Answering the phone is why you're here." It was my job after all.

We started to get callers who were angry.

"Every day I can't get through the line," a contractor complained.

"Did you try calling before or after lunch?" I said

113

politely.

"Look, if I can't get through, you're going to lose business."

"Would you like to talk to Henry now?"

"Yes, I would. Thanks." After a while they stopped complaining. Sometimes I called my father "Dad" at work. I constantly forgot to use his first name.

My father hired a draftsperson. She ate lunch in the office and answered calls when we were out.

My father was an exceptional architect. He knew about a lot of related areas to architecture like millwork, finishes, specifications, construction, permits, and electrical, structural and mechanical engineering. He considered many alternatives when designing a residential or commercial building. He worked hard all day but he also thrived at it because it was his passion.

When I painted, the process was direct, visual, and two-dimensional. I painted to please myself, not anyone else. My father's work had many specifications and by-laws to be met and had to fit the client's needs and budget. As an artist, I used basic design elements but didn't need to deal with the complexity of architecture. Painting was a different type of aesthetic than buildings built ergonomically. Still I learned a lot about design from my father.

"Sandra, what do you think of this?" I leaned over his drafting table at a residential elevation.

"Nice profile with horizontals and clean lines. The chimney and brickwork are nice accents. Why are the windows different sizes? Wouldn't it look better if their heights matched on the outside?"

114

He pulled out a floor plan of the main and upper floor.

I examined the drawings further. "Oh, I see. The smaller window with glass block is for the master bath. And you raised the windowsill there because of the stairwell guardrails. I see form follows function."

My North American Architecture class in university helped me build a vocabulary of building elements. I had learned about famous architects such as Louis Sullivan, Ludwig Mies van der Rhoe, and Frank Lloyd Wright. Sullivan adopted the phrase "form follows function" and made it famous.

Working at the office was educational. When he took on some new projects, my father hired two more draftspersons who were both female. Initially, I intended to only work there temporarily, but years later I was still working in that office. I could have tried to pursue my art but instead I traded in my dream for a regular paycheck.

#

Wanting more variety in my job, I applied at the Vancouver School Board for a supervision aide position. It was a half-day job that would allow me to still work at my father's office during the afternoon. The job consisted of supervising kids at recess and lunch and doing general tasks in between. Initially, I was on call. One of the schools I worked at I liked very much. I applied for a permanent position at an elementary school annex, where the teachers taught students from kindergarten up to grade three.

"I'll come right down to it. Sandra, do you want the job?" The vice principal was a petite lady with white hair. She sat next to me at her office.

"Yes, I certainly would."

"Good. There's just one other thing. Will you mind doing one-on-one with a special needs child for half an hour during lunch while the special education assistant takes her lunch break?"

At that point, I felt cornered. I had just been offered the job and now she wanted me to perform this extra duty not covered by the union contract. If I didn't agree to the extra duty, it would set up a conflict between us. I didn't want to start on bad footing. Also, if I didn't agree, possibly I'd lose the position.

I smiled. "I think I could manage that." So for half an hour every day I worked one-on-one with an eight-year-old girl who couldn't talk and wore diapers. She wore a helmet to protect her head if she fell. She knew some sign language but no one showed me the meaning of her signs. When she looked at books, she tore out the pages. She couldn't write or read.

The union rules stated supervision aides were hired specifically to supervise students. They were not required to do clerical work or work one-on-one with special needs children.

Months later, I wrote a letter to the union to complain about working with the special needs child. I did not have an issue with the girl, but disagreed with the bending of the rules by the vice principal. After a meeting, I won the right to refuse that work but continued to do other duties to fill the time between recess and lunch.

The teachers gave the supervision aides work to do between recess and lunch. The two of us photocopied and collated workbooks for the students. We laminated the students' work and posters which the teachers used to decorate their rooms. I climbed ladders to staple colored paper to bulletin boards and reach high places to help sort through books and supplies.

One day I brought my art portfolio to the studio and showed the staff. One of the teachers said to me, "Would you be interested in participating in an artist series we are doing? We separate two classes into groups of five or six students. Each group studies an artist. Each student does a painting in the artist's style."

"What would you like me to do?"

"We'd like you to be a mystery artist," she said.

I brought a painting to school. The teacher put it on an easel surrounded by a circle of six students and myself.

"This is a painting by a mystery artist. What can you tell me about this artist's work?"

One student looked closely at the signature at the right bottom corner of the painting. "The artist is S. Yuen."

"I saw that too," chirped another student.

"What can you tell me about the style of the painting?" asked the teacher.

A boy with glasses peered closely. "It's very bright and colorful. It's an original."

"What does it mean to be an original?"

"It's not a copy. It's the real thing," he said.

"Who is the portrait of?" the teacher asked.

"It looks like a man like you'd see in a comic book," a blonde girl answered. She was an identical twin in grade two with her sister.

"What do you notice about the background?" asked the teacher.

117

"It's like a window. I can see things in it."

"Like what?"

"Shapes and colors."

"The background is a pattern which is part of the artist's style," clarified the teacher.

"It's a trademark," I said softly.

The students looked at me. The teacher nodded and smiled.

A week later, the students gathered to present information about each artist. One group studied Henri Matisse and presented their artwork done in his style. The palette they used was much like Matisse's. Each group presented their artwork. At the end, my group stood up at the front of the class.

"We studied S. Yuen, a mystery artist. This artist uses bright colors in the foreground and background, and paints people from imagination. Here are the pictures we painted in the style of the mystery artist."

I gasped at the paintings of the students. I saw the bright primary and secondary colors and the bright backgrounds with light and color.

The teacher stepped forward. "The mystery artist we studied is here with us today." The students turned their heads, looking for visitors. "The mystery artist is Sandra." The students were surprised. They weren't familiar with my last name. They cheered and clapped.

"Sandra has painted for nine years. She's educated in the fine arts. We are glad to have her as our mystery artist."

"Can I have your autograph?" asked one student.

"Me too?" said another.

At the following lunch hour, many of the students

approached me, wanting my autograph. One of the staff asked me if I'd like to exhibit in the main hallway at the school. I brought six large paintings to the school and hung them in a corridor. One of the students took my picture next to one painting.

Fame is relative. To me, having seven and eight year olds ask for my autograph was a heartwarming and positive experience. After all, weren't they the driving force of the future?

Wedding Bells

March 1994 - August 1994

For years I had been in love with Greg, but we didn't marry. First I wanted to finish university before I got married. The year I graduated, his father passed away, then his mother died two years later from cancer. He was greatly affected by the loss of his parents. He continued to live in the family home with three of his siblings.

Greg put up with a lot in our relationship but he was always steadfast. Despite my temper tantrums, manic and depressed states, and delusions, he liked me. He didn't complain or treat me badly. He was always just a phone call away. He was constant.

I developed some delusions about Greg's family. He had three brothers and four sisters. I thought I met his extended family in hospital in the early 1980's. I believed they were sent there to help me through a difficult time. Actually, I didn't know his family at that time. Again, it was a fabrication to connect the present with the past. In my mind, all aspects of my life were linked to the past. I tried so hard to make sense of that critical time, it made me desire to hold on to it somehow, as if I could explain it all away, denying I was ever ill. By deceiving myself, I continued to live in a world of fantasy.

I continued working and saw Greg several nights a week and on weekends.

Greg had an interview and was hired to be support staff for the school board. He was also hired as a part-time custodian. Now he was working three jobs, including

120

gardening, plus keeping up other commitments. He was ready to pop the question.

One Saturday, Greg bought lunch and we ate burgers outside on a school bench. It was fairly mild on a breezy afternoon. After he ate his burger, he lay down on the bench and stared up at the sky. I sat next to him, drinking pop with a straw.

"How 'bout it?" he said in the most casual manner.

"What are you talking about?" I licked ketchup off my fingers.

He sat up, smiled, and faced me. "Do you want to get married?"

I could have jumped ten feet in the air. After ten years of dating, he finally popped the question. Suddenly, I was apprehensive. Could we afford a wedding? Could I plan a wedding? He saw the uncertainty in my expression. "Think about it."

The next day I went to see him. "Remember that question you asked me?" I knelt and hugged him around the legs. "The answer is YES!"

We went to the department store. I wanted to hold out for a diamond ring, but he suggested a gold one. He bought me a gold ring with filigree and a heart design. "It's the meaning that counts," he said.

Around the same time, Penny got engaged to her boyfriend Jack. I was thrilled for her. My family gathered for dinner to celebrate their engagement and my mother's birthday. We feasted on roast beef, sticky rice, and vegetables. My grandmother made chow mein.

"I'm so happy for you. I've waited a long time to see

121

you married," my mother said to Penny.

There was a knock at the door. "Who would that be?" I said, with full knowledge of who it was and exactly why he was there.

Jack opened the door and there stood Greg.

"I was just in the neighborhood and decided to drop by." Greg took off his sunglasses.

"C'mon in. Join the party," said the others.

Greg sat down next to me.

"I'm very happy to hear about Penny's engagement but I also have some news," I said.

My mother froze. Silence filled the room.

"Someone else is getting married."

"Who?" Penny asked, wide-eyed with curiosity.

"Greg is getting married." I paused for effect. "And he's getting married to me!"

Around the table, people smiled and cheered. My mother looked shocked.

Po Po smiled broadly. "If I wasn't here I wouldn't know," she said. We all laughed.

Somewhere along the way, my parents realized how much Greg benefited me and how much we cared about each other. They learned to accept him first as my boyfriend then as my life mate. When they got to know his family, they saw the good in them. They knew that if I married Greg, I was also marrying into a stable, supportive family who would take care of me. It wasn't so important that Greg wasn't a Christian; rather it was important that I married the person I loved the most. It was my decision to make, not theirs to choose.

We told Greg's family about our engagement and

they were happy for us too.

So we celebrated at a joint engagement party for Penny, Jack, Greg and myself. We all cut the cake and there was a lot of joy in the house. Penny got married in the spring. Greg and I planned our wedding for August that same year.

#

Greg's home was designed and built by his parents. The house had hardwood floors and two levels. Greg and his siblings ran the family home like a tight ship. Because they had pets, they vacuumed every day. Laundry was done four days a week. Every week they bought groceries.

Greg was always involved in a house project like installing new double-glazed windows, sanding the floor and re-varnishing it, painting, installing laminate flooring, upgrading the electrical system, fixing leaky pipes, replacing old appliances, designing a new porch, and the list goes on.

I always thought Greg's blood and sweat were in his house. He was proud of his handiwork.

One of his brothers, Mel, jokingly called me, Greg's "main squeeze." He laughed at his own joke. Greg's extended family was close and often gathered for birthdays and special occasions.

#

One morning I called my dad at the office to tell him I hadn't slept a wink all night.

"Why don't you take the day off?" he offered.

"The whole day? Sure, thanks dad." I was surprised and pleased at his suggestion. I went downstairs and passed by the laundry room where we have a spare kitchen. There were rows of tart shells sitting on a tray on the table. Ava came out of her bedroom.

"What are the tart shells for? Does mom have a Bible study or something?"

"Oh, I don't know."

Thinking nothing of it, I decided to call Greg and he invited me over. I arrived at his house. I asked his sister Sheila about her plans for the afternoon.

"I'm going to buy a new patio umbrella."

"Right this minute?" I was amused.

"Because you never know when people will come over."

"Are you expecting someone? It's just me here."

I accompanied her to buy a new patio umbrella. They invited me to stay for dinner. After dinner, Greg planned that his brother Mel would take us in his van to pick up a new bed for us. Mel brought Rose, his baby daughter, who was ten months old. We went to a store in Richmond to buy the mattress and box spring. When we returned to the house, Mel parked out back.

"Take Rose and go into the house. We'll take care of the mattress and put it in the basement," said Greg.

So I cradled Rose in my arms and took her up the back steps into the house. Sheila ushered me in and pointed down the hall. I could hear women talking. I looked through the open French doors into the living room. My mom, sisters, aunts and grandmother, and many of Greg's female relatives shouted "Surprise!" I just about dropped the baby.

I was speechless. I had no clue they had planned a surprise bridal shower. The room was decorated in turquoise balloons, paper bells and ribbons. The guests congratulated me. After opening the gifts, we had refreshments including a frosted cake.

"The cake almost didn't make it," remarked Sheila. "It split in half when we brought it in. I made some icing and Penny repaired it."

"How did you prepare so fast?" I asked. "We weren't gone that long."

Mel's wife said, "I was down the street, waiting for you to leave."

"Where did you put all the food?"

"At Gayle's," responded Sheila. I smiled at Gayle, Greg's sister, standing by the doorway. She lived close by.

"How did you find time to decorate?" I asked.

They laughed. I guessed some things should remain a mystery.

#

Greg and I asked his sister Leanne if we could have the wedding in her garden. She and her husband Antonio owned a beautiful house and had a large, landscaped backyard in Richmond.

Antonio confronted me with a stern expression. "You asked my wife, but you didn't ask me."

Worried I had offended him, I said, "May we please have our wedding in your wonderful garden?"

"That's better," he said.

"Is that a yes?" I asked.

He nodded and a sly smile appeared on his face. I didn't need to worry.

We looked up marriage commissioners in Richmond. We made an appointment to see one and

125

arrived at his house on a sunny afternoon. After introductions, Greg and I sat back casually on the couch ready to plan the service. He took one look at us and said, "Are you serious about this? This is a long-term commitment."

Greg and I looked back at him and nodded. I figured he expected us to sit close and hold hands like we were truly in love. We weren't ones to be affectionate in front of strangers. So I moved a little closer to Greg and that seemed to satisfy the marriage commissioner.

Sheila and I had become friends over the years I had visited Greg's house.

"Would you, could you be my maid of honor?" I asked her. She agreed. "It's a big responsibility because I need you to help plan the reception. You'll need a dress and shoes."

She nodded. "Of course, Sandra." I knew she was humoring me. She acted polite and respectful despite my bossy attitude.

I set about sewing my wedding dress out of white lace. Sheila pre-washed the fabric to make her dress. I offered to help her cut it out, but out of eagerness, I botched it up. She had to start all over again, without my interference. I think by the end of it she had attempted three dresses. The final one was turquoise silk with a matching bolero jacket.

Shoes were next. She bought a pair of white ones, which she took to the shoe repair to ask them to dye turquoise for her. The shoes weren't ready on time. After some haggling, they were returned to her but the dye hadn't set properly. When she wore them, the dye rubbed off onto her hosiery.

The other preparations included invitations, renting chairs, tables and umbrellas, decorating and preparing the food. We ordered two fruit-filled cream cakes.

A family friend did the bouquets and other flower arrangements. I chose irises and baby's breath.

The day before the wedding, the wedding party and other helpers gathered at Leanne's house to set up.

"Okay, people. Listen up." I stood on the deck, giving out orders like a lieutenant. "The wedding will take place at one thirty tomorrow. It's going to be sunny and we need to set up the chairs and the tables for the food. Let's get to work."

"Okay, Ms. Dictator," Sheila called out, humoring me again.

We had a brief walk-through. Greg took care of planning the music.

Early the next morning, while I had a leisurely breakfast with my family, Greg's sisters, and other helpers were busy. They gathered at Leanne's house early in the morning to decorate and finish setting up. They decorated the deck with flowers and foliage. A trellis was set up where Greg and I would stand. Sheila and others went back home to change and drove back across the bridge to Richmond again.

It was a sweltering afternoon. Guests arrived early. The guests were well into the soda pop before the wedding began because they were thirsty and it was so hot.

My paternal grandmother, my Ngin Ngin, had a stroke before the wedding and lived at a care facility. On the way to Leanne's, we stopped by the care facility so my mother could give her a rose from the wedding. She got to her room but she was gone.

"Where's Marie?" she asked one of the nurses.

"She's gone to her granddaughter's wedding," she said.

Through her determination, she found a way to make it to the wedding. I was ecstatic.

After we arrived, I stayed upstairs by the window to watch the crowd of eighty guests gather outside. The marriage commissioner, Greg and his best man waited downstairs. The best man was Greg's younger brother. Soon it was time to begin the ceremony.

The guests assembled. Bing Crosby's "Be Careful, It's My Heart" played in the background. The marriage commissioner, Greg and the best man stood in front of the guests. The ring bearer and flower girl soon joined them.

Sheila wanted to wear her sunglasses because the sun was so bright. I refused her request. She walked down the aisle with tears in her eyes not from joy but because of the sunlight. I walked down the aisle with my father.

I like ceremonies to be short and sweet, which it turned out to be. My father gave a touching speech.

Greg and I said our vows and he put the ring on my finger that he had bought me before.

We signed the register and guests took pictures. The service ended and people took to the shade of the trees and umbrellas. Ladies in the kitchen busily heated up chicken wings and appetizers. Sandwiches, fruit, vegetable dips and other foods were served before we cut the cake.

When Sheila took something hot out of the oven, the oil splattered. She ended up with spots of oil on her new silk dress. After all the hard work of making that dress, it was stained. "Maybe it's a sign of good luck," I said.

"Actually, no. I think it's just a stain," she said. "You shouldn't be in the kitchen. Go see your guests."

They shooed me out.

The day after the wedding, Greg and I spent our honeymoon in Parksville. It was blissful. For many years, we returned to Parksville for an annual vacation.

#

There were some real characters in Greg's family. At get-togethers, there was a lot of animated talk and laughter. After living with my biological family since birth, I found I had a whole other family that supported me.

After the wedding, Greg and I lived in his family home, which came as no surprise. I owed a lot to Greg and his family for giving me a caring environment in which to live.

The transition to living in his family home was fairly smooth. I bonded with his siblings and soon I was one of the bunch.

When I grew up, my parents did their best to provide a stable home environment but marrying into Greg's family was another type of life. They treated me like a younger sister. I had few responsibilities in the home. If I couldn't manage cooking, cleaning and work, someone would always pick up the slack. If I wanted company, there was always someone there. If I desired privacy, I could shut the door to our bedroom.

"How do you all get along so well? I think it's remarkable," said my father. "I'm pleased with the way they take care of you."

My parents were both relieved I had finally married. I was happier and more content in my new role. After watching me suffer for so many years, they hoped the worst was over and I would continue in remission of my illness and in good health.

Greg and I occupied a bedroom in the basement with an adjacent room with a television, a computer, a collection of CD's and DVD's, books, and comics. He and I installed parquet flooring. He finished the rooms with pine ceilings and walls. It was quite cozy on cold nights.

Marriage meant so much more to me because we waited so long. I felt secure and loved. From then on, I thought it would be smooth sailing, but I was wrong.

Dealing with Phobias and Deaths in the Family

September 1994 - July 1997

One thing that happens when one develops schizophrenia at a young age is that one becomes frozen in time. The illness may hinder the natural development toward maturity. Periodically, I reverted to the way I felt when I first got ill. I was in a state of self-denial for many years. I couldn't accept the fact that I had a loss, which I'd never get back.

My goals were always about the next step or challenge to gain recognition and approval. I kept achieving because I believed recognition and success would make me a better person.

The drive to succeed left me unsatisfied because I always wanted more. I needed to alter my point of view, but I was preoccupied with the past.

I ruminated continually over past events in my life trying to make sense of my experience. I spent hours reinterpreting past events, and winding fabrications and roundabout explanations for minute details of my life. I'd get angry or sad when I relived those bad experiences in my mind.

The answer was to let the past go. I had to forgive my parents for not being able to identify my problem earlier and myself for not asking for help. At that time, I was too afraid and unsure to tell anyone about the voices and the growing conspiracy concocted in my mind. If my family had been educated or told about schizophrenia and its outward signs like neglected hygiene, social withdrawal, depression, and poverty of speech, perhaps I would have been diagnosed earlier. Perhaps the illness wouldn't have been as severe or prolonged if I received help sooner.

At that time, I had no insight to know I was falling into a pit, digging a hole deeper and deeper until I couldn't climb out.

#

During my life, I developed phobias toward certain things. I had a fear of speaking up in class or in social situations. If I had something to say, my blood pressure would rise, my heart would beat rapidly, and I'd feel flushed and very anxious. To alleviate the discomfort, I had to say something. Sometimes I'd think of something to say but it would be too late.

I feared failure. In the past, I always had to win. If I failed at anything, big or small, I would feel bad about myself even if it wasn't under my control. My competitive nature was so strong that I stopped playing competitive sports, board games, or cards because I disliked losing. After university, I could not tolerate taking credit classes because of my fear of not performing well. Even in non-credit classes, I felt pressure to excel.

Another fear I had was driving to places I didn't know. I would find the address of my destination and prepare a mental map of each street and turn I would make. I had to know precisely where I would park ahead of time. Once parked, I would worry about the time limit on my parking, constantly checking my watch.

I had a fear of falling. Twice I sprained my ankle at the park. I became afraid of walking or running down steep hills.

I was afraid to take risks. If someone asked me to try surfing or skiing, I declined out of fear I'd drown or get injured. I didn't travel out of town alone. I didn't stay out late at night.

If I was invited to an event, I'd get apprehensive and nervous about going alone. Even if Greg accompanied me, I would have difficulty starting conversations with others. I was afraid to try new things or do things that made me feel uncomfortable. I was cautious, unable to take the bull by the horns or be courageous enough to take risks that could have been advantageous to me.

#

The same year I got married, I stopped seeing Dr. Franklin. I was grateful that he helped me through some tough times for over a decade. He saw my progress from finishing school to maintaining a job, but he recognized I still had daily struggles because of stress and sedation. I remember one of the last times I saw him.

"My illness controls me," I said. "Sometimes when I move from reality to delusion, there's a minute period of time where I can see both sides of the fence. I see my family and life as they are, but I also see another parallel world where I am the subject of deception and cruelty. Then I fall deeper into psychosis and lose objectivity. I see no way out of my dilemma. What should I do?"

Dr. Franklin looked at me and said nothing.

"Please help me. Give me advice or a reaction. Say something!"

"You come from a complex place. I can't fix it for you. Our time is up."

133

I left crying. I had to call my mother and Ava to come pick me up because I couldn't drive home. Ava drove my car and my mother chauffeured me home. I decided I wanted to change psychiatrists. Dr. Franklin and I had reached the end of the road.

At the time, I wondered if Dr. Franklin stopped giving me support because he wanted me to see a different psychiatrist. He knew about my rigidity, my unshakeable false belief system, and my lack of logic. He had exhausted all his avenues of ways to help me. He referred me to a mental health team.

I attended my first appointment at a local mental health team. Previously, I was unfamiliar with mental health teams. They serviced a lot of people with varying diagnoses. The team consisted of psychiatrists, case managers, rehabilitation therapists, occupational therapists, nurses, and support staff.

My assessment was quick. I was introduced to Carol, a case manager, and Dr. Sterling. He asked me a battery of questions. After the question period, he relaxed slightly. "You qualify. You will be accepted to the team."

"Who will be my doctor?"

"Who do you think?" he said and left.

Carol and I got along well at first. I was glad to see a female case manager, because I felt she would demonstrate more compassion and empathy toward me. She saw me once a month and offered support and tools to help me cope with stress and problems I experienced. I saw Dr. Sterling once every three months for medication checks. He would ask me to tap my fingers together and stick out my tongue to check for any indication of tardive dyskinesia or other side effects.

It wasn't long before I started to share my frustrations with Carol. I felt stuck between a rock and a hard place. Periodically, I would still deny my illness. "How do I know my paranoia isn't reality-based? Maybe Darren was outside my house." I wanted confirmation.

"Why would he do that?"

"Because he was a troublemaker and wanted to ruin my life, which he continues to do."

"He has no contact with you. You don't even know him."

"He's working with you. You are all in it together." I leaned forward and gripped the arms of my chair.

"No one's after you." Carol shook her head. "Why is any of this important to you now?"

"It means I'm not crazy!" I squeezed my fists with anger. "If it's in my head does that mean it's my fault that I'm ill? I can't win either way."

"You're depressed. That's part of your problem."

"What's the other part?"

"It's time to see Dr. Sterling." She stepped out of the room and returned with reinforcements.

Dr. Sterling sat down in a chair across from me.

"I'm depressed and I can't cope. I'm having obsessive thoughts." I avoided eye contact.

"I'm raising your trifluoperazine dosage." He scribbled on a notepad.

"I get so tired from the meds. Is that the best thing to do?"

"It's the only thing to do."

I got the impression that Dr. Sterling disliked me

135

immensely. He'd never stay in the room with me for over five minutes. I sensed he didn't want to deal with me.

The truth was he treated over a hundred patients. All needed medication checks and time to see him. In the teams, case managers saw the clients as often as needed. The psychiatrists averaged seeing the clients once every three months, relying on the reports of the case managers who would alert them if a crisis arose.

"I hate these pills," I complained. "I think suicide is a good alternative. Maybe if I end it now, you'll all sleep better." I was often flippant or condescending, because of the frustration of having a chronic illness. "Dr. Sterling, you look a little agitated. Are you alright?"

I knew Dr. Sterling was very wise. I also knew he had a lot of insight into my personality and illness. However, he wasn't forthcoming in sharing his insights with me because of my antagonistic, uncooperative manner. He knew I lived behind walls of my own making.

Carol did her best to help me. "You can see the cup as half-empty or half-full. Figure out your values in life and don't pressure yourself to succeed at these enormous tasks you set for yourself. Rome wasn't built in a day. You are very productive most of the time. Invest in stress management. Going to bed early and eating a proper breakfast are ways of taking care of yourself. In the long run, it would be wise to use self-care."

"I'm not into taking long bubble baths or buying bouquets of flowers to brighten up my life. I want to get somewhere, but I'm stuck in dead-end jobs with no future."

"Then quit."

"I can't quit. I need money to live."

"Go on disability."

"Go on disability? After earning a Bachelor's degree and working for years, how can I go on government handouts? I haven't been in the hospital for fifteen years. Does that make sense to you?"

"It will help you cope better."

"Nonsense. I need to work."

"Then change other areas of your life. Are you getting enough exercise?"

Her suggestions were lost on me because of my fixed attitude. My behavior didn't change but continued to be trouble for Carol.

I began to call her "Dr. Carol" as an insult. By giving her that title, it meant I regarded her as my psychiatrist. I felt the prognosis and monthly records of our meetings were in her hands. Dr. Sterling had limited sessions with me, so I believed the person in charge of my case was Carol. She was on the frontline and so my anger was directed at her.

Over several years, my mental health continued to have highs and lows. I regressed into a depressed, angry state. I was demanding and difficult. I believed that during past sessions with Dr. Franklin, he had hypnotized me repeatedly without my knowledge. I believed he was part of the plot against me.

I quit working for the school board and reverted back to working only at my father's office.

I took on more duties over the years as I worked at the office. Most days I came in late. Other days I didn't show up at all. My father was concerned and worried at times. He felt if I kept busy working, I'd put the foreign ideas out of my head. He'd call me at 11 A.M. to say, "Are you alright?"

"I'm not coming in today. I don't feel well."

"If you aren't coming in, call me. I need to know where you are. Otherwise, I don't know what's happening."

"I'm sorry, I can't make it. I'll have the checks made out later this week."

A regular employer wouldn't have condoned my absenteeism, but I guess working for my father involved a certain amount of leeway.

#

I looked forward to Sunday mornings. For many years, my grandmother and I would spend every Sunday morning together. I'd pick up Po Po and take her to restaurants, malls or grocery stores. She would always buy me breakfast. I'd offer to pay but she never let me. I'd carry her bags of groceries when we shopped in Chinatown or grocery stores. When she reached her eighties, she really began to feel her age.

"I'm too old. I'm not happy anymore. I miss your Gung Gung," she said.

"No, Po Po. We all love you. I don't want you to go."

One day she called me to take her to the hospital. I drove to her home. I said, "Do we need to go right away? Are you okay?"

I helped Po Po carry her overnight case to the car and took her into the hospital. Another relative met us there at Po Po's request. I knew Po Po was experiencing symptoms but I didn't know any details. The doctor in emergency checked her vitals. Po Po told me I could go

138

home.

The next day she was discharged and back home. She seemed fine until several months later when she was admitted to the hospital again. I went to visit her.

"Hi, Po Po. How are you feeling?"

"Oh, I'm fine." She smiled. She was always the example of propriety. If anything was wrong, she wasn't one to tell me. "Would you like something to eat? Would you like some peaches?" She pointed to her dinner tray.

I was amused that even though she was in a hospital bed, she still had concern for me. "Oh, no. That's your dinner. I'm going home to eat with Greg."

"I can't eat it all."

I smiled. We visited for a while then I said, "See you tomorrow!" I gave her a hug and waved goodbye.

The next day, my father and Penny came to my home. Penny said, "Po Po passed away. She died from congestive heart failure," Penny said.

The memorial service was at our family church. I had lost my Gung Gung twelve years previously, but it didn't hit me as hard as losing my Po Po. I didn't know how to grieve. I didn't know how I should feel. I couldn't deal with her death.

#

My paternal grandfather, my Ye Ye, developed dementia. He called me from Chinatown, demanding that I come to get him because he bought me a barbequed duck and soy chicken. I refused saying I was too busy at home. He would get awfully mad.

"Call my father. He'll pick you up," I said.

"He won't pick me up. He told me to call you!" he

139

shouted into the phone.

Other times, he'd call the office and say, "My grandson is a millionaire!"

One time I answered the phone. "The doctor gave me IQ pills," he said. "They made my memory improve. I can remember things I couldn't before."

Ye Ye lived in Chinatown. My uncle called him at his apartment for several days and got no answer. He went to his apartment and knocked repeatedly on the door. When there was no answer, he broke the door down. My uncle found Ye Ye lying unconscious on the bathroom floor. The doctor said that he must have fallen about three days earlier.

Ye Ye was revived and admitted to the hospital. He was a proud man. He had little education but worked for years as a hotel and nightclub manager, photographer and salesman. Ngin Ngin and Ye Ye separated when my father was young. She raised eight children with little or no financial support from him.

Throughout Ye Ye's life, he was always concerned about making a good impression. He'd brag about his sons and his own successes.

The last time I saw my Ye Ye, he was lying in a hospital bed. The nurse said that he had passed away in his sleep hours earlier. I wondered if his mind was still able to hear me even though his body no longer functioned.

"Ye Ye, forgive me for not coming to get you in Chinatown. Forgive me for disapproving of you. I love you, Ye Ye," I said to him. After my mother, Ava and I left the room we had to wash our hands to remove any bacteria.

Ye Ye was cremated. Ava sang "Amazing Grace" at

his memorial service. I was supposed to deliver a eulogy, but at the last minute, I decided that I wasn't able to stand up and speak in front of all the mourners. We had a funeral dinner later. I saw my cousins whom I didn't see often. Many of them were married with their own kids. Some couldn't distinguish me from sisters. I didn't know the names of my cousins' children either.

The deaths of my grandparents were very sobering. They made me realize the value of the living. I worried constantly that Greg would die young. This obsession made me fearful and indicated my dependency on him. Dr. Sterling encouraged me not to worry about things outside of my control.

"Everyone dies at some point," he said. "I have every confidence you will recover if and when your spouse dies. Enjoy and appreciate the time you have now. Don't be regretful later."

Relapse

August 1997 - December 1999

During the fall of 1997, I became very depressed. The deaths in my family had affected me strongly. Dr. Sterling tried to increase my trifluoperazine dosage to 20 milligrams, but my condition didn't improve. He prescribed an antidepressant Zoloft, which I took for three days. I developed a burning sensation in my stomach because I was not informed to take the pills with food. I was prescribed ranitidine to relieve my stomach pains. My depression didn't improve so he prescribed valproic acid. I took more time off work but still I didn't improve. Valproic acid is used as a mood stabilizer.

In order to justify the reason I was ill, I believed I was some sort of living martyr saint, who suffered in order to benefit others. I believed the Holy Spirit purified me during a night of fervent prayer. I thought my sacrifices and secret contributions allowed others to rise against their own crises and attain wealth and fame.

At a local restaurant, I had dinner with my parents and sisters. Greg was working and couldn't be there. "I've got something to say." My family was all ears.

"I'm Catholic," I announced.

My parents were staunch Presbyterians. They looked very dismayed. My sisters looked upset.

"How can you be Catholic? We're Presbyterians, Sandra. Suddenly, out of the blue you say this to us?" Ava vocalized my parents' exact thoughts.

"By going to confession, I will be cleansed and

welcomed into heaven," I replied. "I prayed to God for forgiveness. The Holy Spirit took away my angry, critical and jealous nature. I've never felt right about religion until now. I think I'm being called to become Catholic."

"Stop it," my father warned. Other patrons looked curiously at me from other tables. Surely, the waitress could hear me. In obedience, I didn't say anymore.

As we left the restaurant, I took my father's arm and said, "I'm sorry, Dad. I didn't mean to make you angry. But I had this religious experience. At least, I thought I did."

He put his arm around me. "You'll sort it out."

#

In the spring of 1998, I began to feel pressure from all sides, at work and in my personal life. The pressure mounted over several months, until I became very ill and delusional.

I received a mysterious letter from someone who called himself "Robert Montagne" asking me if I owned the Sandra Yuen MacKay Art Gallery in Portland, Oregon. Oddly, the letter had a return address in Strasbourg, France. Flattered, I wrote back that I didn't own the gallery but was an artist and writer working on a screenplay. At the time, I was writing a science fiction story that I wanted to develop into a movie script.

Robert answered back, stating that he knew people in Hollywood who could help me get started.

I was on cloud nine. I did not realize this person was using deception to draw me to him. I thought his name was an alias and in actuality he was Darren from high school. How I made this connection, I don't know. It fed into my false belief system. My preoccupations with him returned.

After all this time, Darren wanted me. I believed he was the son of a famous actor and could help me to become a screenwriter for Hollywood. My obsession led me to act in error and believe the impossible. I sent letters back to him. I was open with Greg about my fascination with this stranger. I was unaware of the amount of Greg's worry and concern.

My regression resulted in Dr. Sterling increasing my trifluoperazine dosage to 25 milligrams. My speech slurred and I walked with my head down. I felt I was trapped in a dense, black cloud. When I drove, I became mesmerized by the steering wheel.

"I think I'm going to have a car accident," I said.

"Then don't drive," Dr. Sterling said. It seemed like a simple solution.

I called my father. "I can't come into work because I can't drive."

"Take the bus."

"There's no point. By the time, I make it there I'll be turning around to come home."

I worked two days out of the week. When I did manage to get to work, my voice slurred and I easily became distracted. I'd mix up my words, which bothered my father. My movements were slow and rigid. I could barely get up in the morning. I was in bad shape.

"I'm prescribing risperidone," Dr. Sterling informed me.

"What's that?"

"It's a new atypical drug. Trifluoperazine can cause tardive dyskinesia whereas risperidone has less of this effect. Cut your trifluoperazine from 20 to 15 to 10 then 5 milligrams. When you are down to 5 milligrams, reduce the dosage to zero and take 1 milligram of risperidone. We will increase the risperidone up to 3 milligrams."

"Is 3 milligrams enough?"

"The strengths of each medication mean different dosage levels have the same effectiveness."

I was glad to go off the trifluoperazine because of the fatigue and stiffness but I was unprepared for the difficult transition from one medication to the other.

Immediately after I began to cut back on the trifluoperazine, my interfering thoughts increased. By the time, I was off trifluoperazine and taking a minimal dosage of risperidone, I was in crisis. My head was dizzy with flashbacks, predictions, information and confusion. I didn't know which way was up. I was in a mental meltdown.

At the office, money was tight. Clients were behind on payments. I had contractors and suppliers calling for monies that the bank account couldn't cover. I worried that my father could barely afford his staff and rent. He took money out of other income to pay payroll and other expenses.

At the same time, I also sought out a new family doctor. I no longer wanted to see my previous family doctor because his secretary left confidential information on our answering machine, which I found very embarrassing. I started seeing a new doctor, which also caused me stress.

She assessed me and asked me to come back the following week.

"How are you today, Sandra?"

"I wish I were someplace else with someone else."

"What do you mean? You're married. Based on what

you've told me, I think you are with the right person." She looked concerned.

"Maybe there's someone better out there. I have a secret admirer who can change my life into something."

"Maybe you are reading something into it that isn't there."

"I hate myself. I wish I weren't here."

"Sandra, I think you need to check in at the hospital."

"Why?" I was surprised.

"I don't trust you can make responsible decisions. Can someone drive you to the hospital?"

"Yeah, but I don't see how a visit to emergency is going to help."

"The only way you are going to get help is to go there."

I went home. "Would anyone like to take me to emergency?" I asked when I got in the door.

A relative drove me to the hospital. After a short wait in emergency, a nurse and doctor assessed me. They checked my blood pressure and asked me a series of questions. The nurse left the room and the doctor stayed to talk to me.

"How do you feel right now," he said.

"Calm and collected," I responded.

"Do you have any psychosis?"

"Right this minute?" I asked. He nodded. I shook my head.

"Are you planning to leave?" he said.

"What do you mean?"

"Your husband."

"Oh, because of the letters I told you about? Not today."

He put down his clipboard. "You are well enough to go home."

"How do you know that? My doctor sent me here."

"You are in control of your senses and are no danger to yourself or others. You don't need to be admitted."

Two weeks later, I hadn't stabilized. I had racing thoughts and visions in my head. Clearly, I couldn't cope. Suspicious and distrustful, I didn't contact Carol or Dr. Sterling at the mental health team.

My family doctor recommended I go back to the hospital. Ava drove Greg and me there. I knew if I exhibited suicidal thoughts or behavior, they would admit me. So when they asked if I felt like harming myself, I said yes. I knew I needed help but I wasn't sure exactly why.

I was admitted to the psychiatric ward in the spring of 1998. By the time I left the emergency room, it was the evening. The evening nurse brought me something to eat. I complained about the graffiti on the wall of my room. I thought it was Satanic. I covered it with a piece of paper held by masking tape. I drew Christ and a cross on the paper with the words "Christ-centered forever."

I had no idea how much my rapid deterioration was affecting my family and Greg in particular. It was a very dark day for him when I was admitted to the hospital.

So I continued in my delusions that my secret admirer was the answer to all my problems. Darren was foremost in my mind. I regressed to the paranoid thinking that I had at fourteen. During a visit from Ava, I talked about leaving Greg and moving to Los Angeles with Robert who I believed was Darren. I was completely entranced by the idea of him. In reality, the sender was a stranger or even a predator.

"I see this is really a serious issue." Ava knew my beliefs were unshakeable in my present condition. "Can I give you some advice?"

I nodded.

"Stay safe until you are capable of making independent decisions that are well thought out and logical."

"Do you think I'm being illogical?"

"I think you are under a lot of pressure. Things are coming at you from all sides. Be with people you can trust."

On the ward, I socialized with the other patients. One showed me how to play poker. I worked on a puzzle with three others. I ordered double portions for lunch and dinner because my medication made me hungry all the time.

One day, my father took time out from his busy schedule to visit me, but he missed me because I was on a group outing to Gastown, a tourist area of Vancouver. The leader of the group looked to me like an actor. I thought his skin was so refined he must have been wearing makeup.

I thought one of the nurses was hypnotizing me at night, asking me questions about terrorist acts in other parts of the world, believing I had the answers to end them.

I believed I was broadcasting my thoughts to people around me. I thought I was to be paid millions of dollars to compensate for being the center of a research study on schizophrenia. If I were an experiment that would explain everything I thought. My deterioration was caused by outside pressure put upon me, in an attempt to burn the illness out of my system. Once cured, I would be famous.

During my hospital stay, I developed the same intense anger I'd had earlier in my illness. I became hostile in a therapy group at the hospital, to the point that the others were afraid I'd lash out at them. I spoke out against Greg in sessions with the nurses, accusing him of pulling the wool over my eyes and destroying my life. In my mind, the one person, whom I loved and depended on the most, became my enemy. Acting out against him was part of the intense rage and paranoia I was experiencing.

The psychiatrist in charge of my case spoke to me in the presence of a nurse. "There's nothing wrong with you. You're going through a transition in your life." I'm uncertain how they arrived at that conclusion. Wasn't my paranoia and anger the tip of the iceberg of a serious psychiatric illness? Did they believe I intended to end my marriage and pursue a relationship with Robert?

My father came again to visit me. This time I was there. He took me for lunch at the University Golf Club. He said, "Sandra, you can do anything. You are the best secretary I ever had. I think you're the best."

"I love you, Dad. You are the best dad I ever had." We laughed.

I was discharged two weeks later. The psychiatrist in charge believed I was not a threat to others or myself, and could work out my problems with Dr. Sterling at the team. Greg and Sheila came to pick me up. Disoriented and confused, I panicked when I got home. Greg seemed alien to me and I had to leave. Flooded with anxiety, I didn't trust him. I called my dad and asked if I could stay at my

Ngin Ngin's condominium, which had no renters at that time. She lived at an extended care unit at the hospital. He agreed. My Aunt Sophie lived in the same building a floor above, so she and my Uncle Blair could take care of me while I stayed there.

Aunt Sophie checked on me often. I felt itchy all the time. I thought the mattress had bed bugs or the shower gel was actually bleach. I tried to shower but I couldn't get rid of the itchiness. I fell and fractured my tailbone. I was constantly hungry and ate continuously.

The first night I stayed there, my Ngin Ngin passed away in the extended care unit. I learned the next day she was gone. We went to see my other aunt, uncle and some of my cousins. My cousin Diane was very close to Ngin Ngin. I helped her organize her thoughts in a eulogy. I offered to deliver it at the funeral. I went home and practiced reading it. I spoke on Diane's behalf at the funeral.

One night, I looked up from washing the dishes and saw a menacing red and black face hovering in front of me. I thought it was Satan. I prayed to send him away. I tried not to be afraid. He lingered then disappeared. I thought my visions must be delusions. My mind was out of balance with all the turmoil of the past few months.

One night, I thought the ghost of Ye Ye was in the room. He was coming to get Ngin Ngin. I felt the presence of my grandmother who told him to stay away. He wouldn't leave. In my delusion, she got angry and told him repeatedly to go away. After a difficult marriage and separation, Ngin Ngin had nothing to say to him even in death, I thought.

Soon I sensed many spirits in the room. I was so

150

frightened I couldn't sleep. I thought there was evil hiding in the closets. At midnight, I went upstairs and knocked on my aunt's door. I spent the night on their couch, sleeping in my robe, nightgown and slippers.

Such bizarre perceptions demonstrated my psychological imbalance, but because of my lack of insight, I couldn't control my thinking.

Uncle Blair took me for long walks downtown and around Granville Island. He was good company. Some other extended family members paid me a visit.

My Uncle Tim and I stood on the balcony of the condo. We had a view of the sailboats and False Creek.

"What are you going to do?" he asked.

I felt the wind on my face. The light was beginning to fade. "Don't you think this would be a great painting studio? I could stand here and paint all day as the light changes over the buildings and the water. I really think this is a special place. If only I could afford to paint all day."

"You are going to keep doing your art regardless?"

"That's all I can do or want to do. Dad's office won't be around forever. I doubt I can find another job because of my absenteeism."

"Money isn't everything to you, is it?" he said. "You're a free spirit."

I received a letter from Robert. I had sent him my temporary address. His letter sat unopened for about a week because I didn't check the mailbox. He wrote in large capital letters, "I spent two hundred dollars a day waiting for you at the Travelodge. I wrote and called you numerous times. I'm leaving tonight. The next step is up to you." I had never spoken to him on the phone. I wondered if he had called the house or office when I wasn't there and others had intercepted the calls. I found the letter to be threatening.

As the days passed, I became lonely and longed for Greg. I called him several times a day. He came and stayed with me overnight. A few weeks later, my father called to say, "The suite is being rented out. You have to leave."

I decided to go home to Greg. He was relieved I was home, but I'm sure he had grave concerns about my instability. Our marriage bonds had never been questioned in the years we'd been married.

The letters from Robert had let my mind wander. I was unsatisfied and dreamed of fairytale romances. I didn't realize how my behavior affected Greg. He remained constant and forgiving. He welcomed me back without punishment or accusations. Later, I found the letters and destroyed them. I never met Robert in person and wouldn't recognize him if I saw him.

#

I met with Dr. Sterling. "I'm angry at all of you. It's your fault that after fifteen years of going to school and working, I ended up back in the hospital."

He flipped through my file and said nothing.

"You gave me so many medication changes, my body couldn't tolerate them all. Now you say I have a schizoaffective disorder? I'm worse off now than I've ever been."

"This isn't new. You have always had a mood component to your illness," he said.

I felt like I was back at square one. Having a schizoaffective disorder meant my symptoms of psychosis and a mood disorder were equally apparent. When I looked back on my mood swings from my teenage years on, it could have been possible I had depression and mania from the start; hence the diagnosis was correct but I didn't want to admit it.

"You took advantage of me and experimented on me!" I lashed out like a caged animal. My face was red with resentment. "You directed my father to apply extreme pressure on me at work and instructed Darren to send me letters. You knew letters from Darren would put me over the edge. You wanted to try to burn the illness out of me."

I believed others were once again plotting against me. Realistically, it was unethical for psychiatrists to cause a patient to become ill, but I wasn't able to see things logically. I had lost the insight that I had before.

"Experimented on you?" Dr. Sterling looked furious. "That's not true! We know you. We know what you're like."

I glared at him in disbelief. "How can you know me if you never see me for more than five minutes every three months?"

"That's it. You're certifiable."

"I want a new psychiatrist and a new case manager." Certainly, I had rights. I felt pinned to the wall.

"If you go that route, you will have to attend a different team. Your home address falls in a different catchment area."

"I can't stay here and I don't want to go there." I felt trapped.

"You can't keep rejecting people. You continue to run away from your problems. I suggest you stay here."

153

Running out of options, I suggested another avenue. "Okay, will you continue as my psychiatrist if I can get a new case manager?" I had some serious issues with Carol. I blamed her for the mismanagement of my case. I wondered if her negligence in my care was part of the ploy to make me hit rock bottom.

"I'll ask if you can see Kathy."

"What are her qualifications?" I worried that she wouldn't be able to advise me on my complex problems.

Dr. Sterling didn't answer but instead left the room. He came back momentarily. "You can see Kathy but if your behavior is like this again, we will deny you services."

Defeated and doubtful, I met with Kathy. "Do you think Carol was out of line in her treatment of me?" I asked.

"Carol is good at her job and she's also my friend. I do not feel comfortable talking about her with you. All I can say is, you can't act the way you did without consequence. You had a part in that relationship. You stopped seeing her."

"I didn't trust her."

"I can see that."

Despite initial tensions between us, I built trust and respect with Kathy. She listened to me at my worst and my best. She had ready advice, which I tried to incorporate into my daily life. She helped me to deal with problems when I was disappointed, fearful or angry.

I dropped the issue of Carol. I would see Carol in the halls or waiting area and I'd say hello or wave. I forgave Carol for any wrongdoing on her part. When I stopped keeping appointments, Carol couldn't help me. I remember she tried to call me at my father's office during my last crisis, but I was already past the point of no return. I had been difficult but felt she had failed me. She did not give me guidance with complex issues like grieving the death of my grandparents. On the other hand, I was unable to heed the advice she did give, because of my hostile, paranoid state.

Dr. Sterling put me on another atypical, olanzapine, and an anti-anxiety medication, clonazepam. He told me that olanzapine could cause weight gain and recommended I exercise to relieve my anxiety and anger as well as prevent excessive weight gain. I started to visit the YMCA three mornings a week. I swam, used weights and the elliptical machine. I did put on some weight but it was mostly muscle. The exercise did help me psychologically. I felt good after a workout. After a year, I was steadily putting on weight and eating more than usual to keep up with my exercise program. It became counterproductive so I canceled my membership.

Kathy suggested I join some of the groups offered at the team. The first one I took was on anger management. I learned the triggers for my anger such as feelings of rejection, unfairness, or failure. Even though current events triggered my anger, they potentially could ignite past emotions. We talked about repression from unresolved problems in my past. I needed to learn how to change my behavior, react in a healthy matter and stop the vicious cycle of my anger. I learned coping strategies to prevent anger from growing. Exercise, journaling and expressing myself through art were some helpful suggestions.

"Why do I get so out of control?" I asked.

"What triggers you?" said the leader of the group.

"Everything."

"Be specific."

"When I see someone who has it too easy."

"You blame them for something that is outside their control. Learn empathy and compassion. Relax, count to ten and use deep breathing. See yourself as that person. Be conscious of how that person feels."

"I develop tunnel vision. I can't see past the red."

"Find ways to break the anger cycle to prevent it before it gets out of control. Are you angry at yourself?"

"I feel I'm a failure. I dislike who I am."

"Do you blame yourself for how you are?"

I nodded.

"It's not your fault that you have an illness, but you can make changes to improve how you manage your illness."

"I feel I'm a bad person."

"Use positive self-talk."

After that session ended, I joined another group to learn about recovery. We talked about elements of recovery including hope, determination, empowerment, meaning, and quality of life.

"Take an active role in all areas of your health. It's your responsibility," said the facilitator.

"What if I can't get out of bed and feel lousy?" I asked.

"At some point, most people feel that way. It's up to you to choose activities to help yourself. Get enough sleep, go for a walk, and make some friends. Those are the kinds of things we are talking about."

In a meeting with Kathy, I talked about finding

156

something to do with my time that fit into the recovery themes I learned in the group. "I suggest you speak with Betty. She can help you find some activities you might like to try."

"I'll do that."

Betty, who worked at the mental health team, asked me some questions and invited me to join an introductory fitness course with other clients. A group of us met once a week for eight weeks. Each time we received instruction on a different activity. We walked, used weights, played badminton and tried yoga. Most of the people in the group were overweight. I think a lot of our weight problems were caused by the medications we took. We were all in the same boat.

After the eight weeks were over, Kathy remarked to me, "You seem emotionally more stable now. Why is that?"

"I feel I'm improving but at a snail's pace. Can't I go faster?"

Creativity, Coping, Strategies, and Ideations

January 2000 - December 2003

At the team, I saw a poster about The Art Studios. "What's The Art Studios? Is that something I would be interested in?" I asked Kathy.

"Are you wanting to take art classes?" she answered.

"I've taken a lot of art classes but I haven't been creative for a long time. I'm rusty."

Kathy smiled. "I think you should try." The Art Studios was a rehabilitation program that offered art classes to people with mental health conditions, funded by Vancouver Coastal Health. Most of the instructors were persons who had mental illnesses with experience or education in fine arts. Members had the opportunity to not only learn creative skills, but also to socialize, volunteer, lead, teach, and sell their work at semi-annual sales.

I got an appointment to be assessed to see if I was suitable to take classes at The Art Studios. I was given an orientation. They offered pottery, sculpture, painting, drawing, and writing classes. I signed up for a drawing class. It wasn't long before I got to know some people. In my college and university days, I had almost no contact with anyone who had a mental illness. After attending the group therapy sessions at the team and once I began attending the drawing class, I experienced a shift. I found out that I wasn't as abnormal as I thought. I met other people with mental illness and suddenly I wasn't alone but part of a community.

I enjoyed the drawing class. We drew still lifes and portraits of each other. Some of the other students complimented me on my ability to draw. When I ran into a few of them again years later, they smiled and said they remembered me from that class.

The instructor encouraged all the students. One student said to the instructor after a demonstration, "You are talented."

The instructor smiled and said, "Sandra is the one to watch."

Inspired, I reawakened my creativity after years of clerical work.

After the drawing class was over, I joined the writing group. The instructor was a blonde woman named Ashley. She gave us ideas and exercises to get us to write. Some people in the group wrote about very painful experiences and emotions. Some of the writing was very original and poetic.

Ashley asked me for coffee one day. We started to email and get together for a walk, swim, or sushi lunch. She was a very talented artist and writer.

Because she was the only friend that I had in a long while, I put a large emotional stake in that relationship. She introduced me to a Vancouver-based art magazine that eventually published my writing. She introduced me to some of her other friends and invited me to her birthday party.

Then one day, out of the blue, she said that she was returning back east. I was distraught, unable to deal with the loss of a friend. I was angry because I didn't know why she suddenly wanted to leave. I wondered if I'd done something to offend her. I emailed but lost touch with her.

The best thing I could have done was to let it go, but I kept hoping we could be friends again. Later, we reconnected and exchanged letters.

The Art Studios had a winter sale. It was crowded with so many buyers and sellers. The mood was exciting and fun. I sold handmade fake fur hats and showcased my portfolio. It was enjoyable to be part of that sale. I laughed and joked in a social atmosphere, which didn't happen often.

Another good thing that came out of joining The Art Studios was that I made some contacts. A group of five female artists including myself put together a group show at Gallery Gachet, a gallery that exhibits outsider art, community art projects, and contemporary art by mentally ill people. We called our exhibition "The Women's Room." I was very excited about being part of that show, which included eleven of my paintings.

#

I asked if I could join a wellness group at the mental health team. We met every Wednesday afternoon and discussed how our lives were going. At first, I said very little and kept my gaze on the carpet. I sat with my arms folded, not wanting to share or respond to others in the group. One member of the group noticed how tense I was. He thought I had a huge chip on my shoulder from the beginning. My contributions to the group were mainly short, brief complaints about my situation. I'd repeat the same problems each week with little variation. I was inflexible, unable to move forward.

"You have a Bachelor's degree?" asked a woman in

the group. "In what?"

"I majored in Western art history but I wasn't a very good student," I replied.

"You're an artist? I wish I could draw or paint," remarked another.

"My art's okay, but it's not good enough," I said. "No one really wants to buy my style of art."

"Why are you so negative about any positive feedback you get?" the facilitator interjected. "You make excuses and refuse to accept a supportive compliment from people who take interest in you. Why is that?"

"Because I'm not a good person and anything I do isn't good enough either."

"Good enough for whom? You are setting yourself up for disappointment. Step back and look at yourself. When you look in the mirror, what do you see?"

"An ugly, fat, stupid person with high ideals who will never measure up."

"You aren't in a competition. Accept yourself and take pride in your accomplishments. I don't mean having boastful pride, but acknowledging yourself. The next time someone says something kind to you, hold onto that emotion and that warm, fuzzy feeling. That's the beginning of gaining confidence in yourself."

I shared my worries and inner demons with the group. I was a perfectionist who never settled for less. I was fixed in my views and unyielding in my relationships with others. This attitude didn't help my situation. No one wants to be friends with an icicle like I had become.

My depression affected my perspective. One day I spoke with Greg. "Why don't you throw me out?" I was upset. "I'm a liability to you and your family. Maybe it's best if you get rid of me and marry someone else who is easier to get along with and can raise children. Don't you want to have children?"

"Sandra, you are most important to me. I think the priority is that you are taken care of and not burdened. My concern for you is stronger than the desire to have children. If you aren't well, a child won't make it any better."

Greg was a wise man. He saw me clear as day. He knew my strengths and weaknesses, and the cycles I experienced as an ill person which were worsened by my futile attitude. Greg dealt with my tirades by trying to placate me as best he could. I never knew how he dealt with the negative energy I flung at him. I thought perhaps he confided in his sister Sheila about me or he directed that energy toward constructive work. He did a lot of physical work to maintain and improve the house and garden and in his jobs.

All my life I wanted to be loved and feel important, and he fulfilled both those wishes.

He knew my illness was chronic which meant I still would continue to experience psychosis or depression at times. He genuinely cared enough to see me through the hard times, and be happy for the days or weeks when I was well and equal in our marriage.

Winter was harder than summer. In the winter, I was inactive, overate and slept a lot. Because I was sluggish, I felt miserable. When spring came, I would go outdoors more and get that precious Vitamin D. In times of idleness, I regressed into delusions and my emotions would spike.

Dr. Sterling asked me, "What comes first, the

emotion or the thoughts?"

"The thoughts set me off."

"Can you change the subject you are thinking about or distract yourself?"

"No, I can't."

"Try to talk your way out of it in your head. Find a way to avoid those troubling thoughts. Think about a person or experience that makes you feel better about yourself."

"When I have these thoughts, they are so real. I can't stop from spiraling."

"You know from past experiences, that every time you follow that way of thinking, you hit a low. By breaking the cycle, you regain control." Dr. Sterling made a note on his pad. "What are your early signs?"

"Fatigue or stress. Sometimes it's like being in a pressure cooker. Over a week or two, my anxiety and worries build until the lid pops off from the pressure bottled inside my body."

"What can you do to reduce fatigue or stress?"

"Get enough sleep."

"You have to learn to relieve your stress by taking breaks and not planning too many activities each day."

#

I had a new family doctor, Dr. Nichol who had some good advice. I spoke to him about my weight gain.

"Don't worry too much about the body mass index. I think it's more important that you feel good about yourself and your health," said Dr. Nichol.

"I'm heavier than I've ever been. I'm concerned about my physical health."

"There are two things you can do. Olanzapine may cause high triglycerides, cholesterol problems, and diabetes. Taking salmon oil capsules will help lower your triglycerides and aid digestion. Exercise will also help you. How about exercise to shed those extra pounds?"

"I used to work out at the gym but I didn't lose weight." I hedged but then said, "I like to walk."

"Why don't you set a goal to walk forty minutes everyday?"

I agreed and started a walking routine rain or shine. I didn't lose weight but controlled myself from gaining more. I usually walked on my own through the cemetery. From there, one could see the mountains, and enjoy the greenery and fresh air. I didn't really associate the cemetery with sadness or grieving. During the day, it was a nice place to walk.

Walking was good in some ways but the problem was I would disappear into my head when I walked. I'd talk aloud to myself, dreaming up some strange ideas. I thought that I could hear relatives talking about me. These weren't auditory hallucinations but paranoid beliefs that I could telepathically hear people talking about me. Sometimes I would shout or swear loudly, believing my voice would broadcast to others miles away.

I kept up my walking routine for about a year. My feet started to hurt when I walked so I stopped walking as often. As a result, I put on weight again. I didn't monitor my diet and any exercise I did was sporadic. Repeatedly, my case manager and doctors told me I had to make lifestyle changes gradually by limiting portions of food, and staying away from excess sugar and fats. They told me exercise was also something I should do regularly not just for my physical body, but my psychological well-being.

Kathy suggested yoga or meditation but I wasn't too interested; however, I know some people that say those activities help to center them and alleviate stress. She also talked about mindfulness, which is described as an awareness of one's actions, feelings, and environment in a patient, non-judgmental fashion. Focusing on breathing or concentrating on a particular activity are ways of staying in the present.

#

I involved myself in sewing projects. I sewed wool coats, pajamas, dresses, pants, blouses, skorts, shorts, polar fleece vests and jackets, hats, curtains, children's wear, duvet covers, pillow shams, tablecloths, and swimming suits. In one year, I averaged one item every two or three weeks. My closet bulged with so many garments. I also sewed a lot for other people.

Sometimes when I sewed, I'd fantasize that sewing for others was a spiritual endeavor. By sewing clothes, I was giving to others not only a service, but also a spiritual offering of good will. If something needed mending, my sewing not only fixed the garment, but also healed that person in some small way. I named these activities as sewing a "wor" which was my own fictitious term meaning a blessing or gift to the recipient. I believed a wor could heal emotional suffering or to help alleviate problems that person was experiencing.

I identified myself to be like Mother Teresa or a messenger of peace or good will. I felt because I had suffered, I was somehow endowed with the power to heal. I believed I was touched by God in some way.

I was very leery of cults. I feared if I were ever drawn into a cult, it would consume me. I am very susceptible to the power of suggestion. Under the influence of a cult or group, I would become dependent on the leader of that group and lose the power to make logical, independent decisions.

I viewed church in the same way. If I went to church, worshiped and became involved in Bible studies or fellowship, I would become enslaved to their religious philosophies.

The danger was that if I prayed or worshiped God, I was susceptible to delusions about possessing spiritual power and believing I was a deity of some type. I would believe God spoke to me and directed me to do things.

The last thing I wanted to hear was that I was a sinner and that I would go to hell if I didn't accept Jesus Christ. I felt it was like a threat not a promise of salvation. Also, if I confessed my sins and became a Christian and subsequently left the church, God would punish me.

Attending Sunday Services disturbed me. I didn't want to be there because I associated the church with punishment from God and being unworthy of God's love.

Because of these barriers, I could not be confirmed in my church or even attend on holidays. It wasn't for me.

Some of my Christian friends and family invited me to functions but I said no. They wished for me to feel God's love and be part of the church community, but I shied away. I did attend a few services, but I would cry when we sang hymns. My doubts and pain rose to the surface and all I could do was cry. After that, I didn't go back.

My father knew I wouldn't listen to him about going to church. He asked an elder to talk to me. The elder joined us for coffee at the mall. He said, "You are part of God's family. You should be with your family."

"I can't reconcile God's love with human suffering," I said. "I feel like I'm being punished for something I didn't do. Greg's family is my family."

On the one hand, I believed I was a healer of mankind but in reality, I rejected the church. It seems contradictory but the delusion that I was spiritually endowed was perhaps a response to the lack of spirituality in my real life. The idea of being a living saint faded when I stopped sewing for a while. I think the associations in my mind happened mainly when I spent time alone at the sewing machine or on walks.

New Insights, Opportunities, and Sorrow

January 2004 - May 2005

Drumming my fingers on a Styrofoam cup, I waited impatiently at the mental health team to see Dr. Sterling. My feet tapped to the beat of a silent band. I rehearsed my words ahead of time. Going to see Dr. Sterling was like a test that I had to pass. If I failed, it might result in an increase in medication. He pushed me to the limit because he knew I was capable and intelligent. Sometimes he spoke very little, but I could envision the wheels turning in his head when I discussed my mental condition and extreme emotional outbreaks.

Despite recognizing the pitfalls of my bizarre notions, I still couldn't shake my preoccupations. Weren't those my lyrics in that song? Wasn't that movie plot something I imagined before? Wasn't I responsible for a career of a director, writer, singer or actor because I had given them my ideas and predicted their success in the present? Starstruck by celebrities, I wanted it all.

In my delusions, others were impressed with my vocal range as a closet karaoke singer. Cameras and microphones recorded my singing in preparation for my exposé when the truth would be revealed.

I would be recognized as the center of the entertainment world.

I had to wait twenty minutes to see Kathy and Dr. Sterling. I stared at the bulletin board. Microwave popcorn sat on a bowl on the table. Clerks marked time typing out reports and notes from meetings. I watched the clock as the

168

minute hand passed the three.

Finally, Kathy appeared smiling and escorted me into Dr. Sterling's office. He swiveled in his chair and posed the question, "How are you?"

"Oh, I'm fine. I did a painting this week. Also I've been going to wellness group. I meet with friends from the group for coffee on Saturday mornings. My mood has been fairly good." I always started with the good things in my daily life to make a favorable impression.

"Are you having symptoms?" He folded his hands in a temple.

I braced myself. I could have said, "I won a million dollars" and he would still respond by asking about my symptoms. "Back up. Did you hear the things I said? Can't you just say, 'that's good' or acknowledge how well I'm doing?"

"That goes without saying. Know it within yourself without continual reinforcement from others."

"I feel trapped like I'll never get anywhere. Why is everything an effort for me? I try so hard, but the road is too long and steep. I can't keep up."

"You're being hard on yourself. You have a lot of strengths. Can you tell yourself differently?"

"What do you mean?"

"Say to yourself, 'I'm going to be gentler on myself. I'm going to do my best based on the time and energy I have.'"

"I feel like I'm the bottom of the barrel. Life is passing me by."

"Why do you feel that way? Appreciate that others are equal to you not less or more. Address your problems

169

and solve them on your own. It's not up to Greg or anyone else to fix things for you."

I resisted the temptation to lie. "I'm having some visions of the future. I think Greg's going to die young." I bit my lip. "I stopped taking my pills." The words tumbled out. "I wanted to see if I could do without them."

"And what happened?" He knew the way the conversation was heading.

"I blew up and had a fight with Greg. I spend more time thinking than anything else."

"If you want to stabilize, take the pills as prescribed," he stated.

"It's my body. Isn't it my right to not take the medication?" I challenged.

"If you refuse medication, we can't treat you."

Kathy nodded in agreement.

"You'd shut the door on me if I don't comply? Isn't it your job to help me?" I said.

"Only if you're willing," he said.

"What if I get a new psychiatrist?"

"Are you certain?" he said. "You would be put on a waiting list. It could take up to six months."

"I'd have to wait that long?" I backpedaled. The muscles in my stomach tightened. Feeling weak, I slumped in my chair. My eyes started to tear. Kathy handed me a tissue.

"Seeing another doctor isn't going to help. You can't keep running away from your problems. Stop running and work with it," said Dr. Sterling. "If you want to reduce your medication, do it with us, not on your own."

"If I go back on, can I take half a dose?"

"That won't be enough to sustain you. You need to take twenty milligrams a day," said Dr. Sterling.

"But I was doing so well."

"The medication was helping. That's why you stabilized. If it isn't broken, don't fix it. Why change the dosage if things are working out?" He reached for his notepad and scribbled down some notes.

"Are you going to go back on your medication?" asked Kathy.

I dug the toe of my shoe into the carpet. Without raising my head an inch, I murmured, "I don't want to take the pills."

"Why?" asked Kathy.

"Because if I take them, it means I'm weak and unable to manage my illness."

"If you were diabetic, would you take insulin?"

I nodded.

"It's no different than olanzapine. There's nothing wrong with taking the medication. It doesn't mean you're weak," Kathy reasoned.

"I know. It's a chemical imbalance," I said.

I took the elevator down alone, feeling lost as a sheep without a shepherd. I clutched an appointment slip for the next visit. At least he heard me. I had tried to go off and failed. I knew deep inside he was right. I needed to stay on the medication even in times of wellness. Still I felt it was necessary to go off the medication to test my ability to cope on my own. The doors slid open. I walked out of the building to a chilly afternoon.

#

Over time, I learned more about ways to manage my

illness. Dr. Sterling told me to look for three things: all or nothing thinking, "futurizing," and comparison.

All or nothing thinking meant I thought in absolutes. Certain days I saw as all negative, even if ninety percent of the day went well.

I saw everything as not good enough. I would say words like "never," "I can't" or "I won't." Because of depression, I was disgruntled and discontent.

Futurizing referred to the belief that I could predict the future. I constantly worried about the future, filling my head with good and bad scenarios of how life would work out. I worried that if Greg died, I would have to forage on my own. I worried that my younger sister would have a car accident or my older sister would become ill. Because I spent so much time obsessing, I spent less time in the present and became emotionally unstable.

Comparison was a big problem for me. "Comparing yourself with others will always end with you not measuring up. That's how comparison affects you," Dr. Sterling warned.

I constantly compared myself to people, who weren't faced with mental illness, had professional jobs and high incomes. They had affluence and monetary success. Their children excelled in school and were also destined for greatness. Feelings of jealousy led me to criticize others. In retrospect, if I had focused less on the faults of others and stopped envying their lifestyle, wealth or prestige, I think I would have grown three inches taller.

"There's nothing wrong with you. Just forget about the past and you'll be fine," others said. Unfortunately with mental illness, that advice didn't always work.

My psychiatrist had more insights. "Your grandiose delusions about your ability overcompensate for the low self-esteem that you had before you got ill. Find some middle ground. You aren't a genius or a saint, but you aren't the bottom of the heap either. Teach yourself to absorb the messages that others are sending you. To function well, try to level out and gain confidence or you will never reach equilibrium. Part of maturity is to know yourself. Constant approval from others shouldn't be necessary. Believe in yourself and in the decisions you make."

"I can do that?"

"As an adult, you have to let go of traits that impede you. You have the ability to change your behavior. Once you do that, your life will change with you."

"I can't believe I'm going to wake up one day and feel relief from the daily struggles I face."

"I'm not saying it's an easy thing. Make steps in the right direction that will stop you from moving in circles and lead you to freedom from excuses."

"What do you mean by excuses?"

"By denying your talents and abilities and shoving them under the rug, you are denying yourself the chance to be free and happy. How can you live well without enjoying life's offerings? Instead, you stay behind a barrier never venturing out to sense the joy and happiness you could have."

"Is it my fault I don't have a rich life?"

"Fault isn't the word I'm looking for. Attitude is a better word."

"So by changing my attitude, I can reach my

dreams?"

"Not necessarily. But trying doesn't hurt."

I went home and thought about Dr. Sterling's insights. Was I really that unforgiving of myself? Was I really so caught up in refusing to engage life?

#

The Art Studios relocated to Victoria Drive. I signed up for a few classes. The renovated building had three studios, offices, and a computer room. The Art Studios was a safe, friendly place. Even though, it ran on a tight budget, it was very successful in helping people like me.

I took a beginner's acrylic painting class. The instructor had a good sense of humor and kept the students entertained. We did some drawing studies before we painted. By studying light, shadow, texture, and perspective, we could better understand the same elements of design in a painting project. I painted a hummingbird and flowers as my first project. I spent a long time on the petals, making each one appear three-dimensional. The instructor told me to use the paint at high viscosity and not water it down. He showed me blending techniques and which colors to mix to create highlights and depth.

One of my iris paintings was purchased and given to the President and Chief Executive Officer of Vancouver Coastal Health at a fundraiser.

I also took printmaking class. I made linocut greeting cards and prints. I sold my linocut cards at The Art Studios sales for three or four dollars each. A real bargain!

I also took intermediate drawing. We worked with charcoal on paper clipped to boards on easels. We worked from a model, drawing quick gesture drawings. One girl

174

who never had training in art found she could draw very well and was pleased with her work. A lot of the students were very talented and we supported one another.

The next class I took was intermediate painting. The instructor was an expert on color, depth, composition and perspective. When we painted still lifes, he'd point out areas in which I could improve. I found the instruction at The Art Studios to be on par with the colleges I had attended.

The instructors at the studio were knowledgeable and encouraged the students to do their best. Art is therapeutic, because it allows one to use one's hands to create objects in clay or with paint or charcoal and results come very quickly. The creative process frees the mind, and allows one to explore and focus on something fun and interesting.

A rehabilitation assistant informed me about a job opportunity with the Traveling Art Show, which exhibited works by The Art Studios members at various locations in Vancouver. I applied, was interviewed, and hired as an assistant. It was my job to drive to various venues with a staff member and a trunk loaded with artwork. Together, we transported and hung the paintings or displayed ceramic work. Each piece was labeled with the artist's name, title of piece, medium and price. Sometimes work sold and other times people said how much they enjoyed having the art at their workplace. The Traveling Art Show aided members in marketing their work outside of the studio.

A month later, I got a call from The Art Studios coordinator. "Sandra, I heard you are a good writer. Our writing instructor is unable to teach the class. It's supposed to start next week. Would you be willing to take on the class?"

"I signed up to take that class. How do you know I can write?" I was published in various magazines at the time but didn't remember sharing that information with her.

"We know you. If you are willing, we'll waive the interview. Can you start next week?"

So I was hired to teach creative writing for a year. I put together a course outline. I planned lessons on poetry, settings, plot structure, character development, and point of view. Each class we did some fun exercises.

"It was a dark and stormy night. Use that phrase in a story," I instructed the students. After ten minutes, they would read their writing aloud and get constructive feedback. "Use at least three senses in describing a setting," I asked. Each exercise taught something new. "Write a poem about an emotion" was another exercise. Teaching was a challenge but I enjoyed it.

#

Many of my relatives had children. Kids were everywhere I looked. When I reached thirty-nine, I reconsidered if Greg and I had made the right decision not to have children. I talked to Greg again.

"Many couples don't have children. It's not a necessity," he said. "You're free, Sandra. You paint and write. You don't have that added responsibility. You are a good aunt to your nieces and nephews."

"But don't you wonder what it would be like to have our own child?"

176

"No, I don't," he replied. "You're my prime consideration." He worked with children in his job and was a good uncle. Greg had other reasons why having children wasn't the best idea. "Most of the time you are fine, Sandra. But sometimes something clicks in your mind and you become a different person. You switch like night and day. It's not you."

I spoke to Kathy and Dr. Sterling at the mental health team. "I'm considering having a child. I'm almost forty. I may not have another chance."

"What's changed that you want to have a child?" questioned Kathy.

"I feel I've missed the boat. My relatives have kids." I'd never shown an interest in child rearing or even babysitting. But wouldn't having a child make my life more meaningful?

"Having a child isn't going to make you more important as a person. Plus you will have added responsibility. If you are going to have a child, do it for the right reasons. It changes your whole life."

"Would I pass on schizophrenic genes to my child? I don't think I can raise a child but I think about it."

"You don't have to conform to traditional roles," advised Dr. Sterling. "Find things to do, make friends, work or volunteer. Live your own life. Don't compare yourself with others. That will only give you more problems. Instead, think of the activities you can do, not the business of others. Find your own role and identity as an individual."

Self-affirmations repeated daily, or when I felt disappointment, helped me to rebalance. Instead of thinking others had more than me or better circumstances, I gradually learned to like and appreciate Sandra. So when I felt inadequate, I said to myself, "I'm Sandra. I'm a writer and an artist. I'm creative. I'm human. I can get through this."

I was fortunate to have an understanding and compassionate partner. Greg and other family members took care of me despite my complaints and symptomatic behavior.

#

I was in a drawing class at The Art Studios one morning, when my sister Ava came into the studio with her husband Lee.

"Hi! How did you know I was here?" I was surprised.

"I'm a social worker. Of course I know where you are," she jested. "Come to the car with us." She led me out the door and down the street. I sensed something was wrong.

"Is it mom?"

"Wait until we get to the car." She unlocked the car door and sat me down in the passenger seat. "Dad died this morning."

I wailed and tears poured down my cheeks. Ava and Lee cried with me. I couldn't believe he was gone. It was like someone had put a knife in me. "How did he die?"

"They say he had an aneurism. A blood vessel broke in his brain and blood went into his brain. It was unpreventable. The walls of the vessel may have become thin with age."

She hugged me. She drove me to mom's while Lee

took my car and went to pick up Greg to meet us there.

When we got there, I saw the coroner's car parked out front, ready to take dad away.

When I went inside, my mom hugged me. "I wanted you to see dad before they took him away," she said. "I told them to wait."

Ava held my arm as I looked in the master bedroom and saw dad on the bed. The drapes were drawn. The quilt covered his body; only his face and shoulders were visible. He looked peaceful like he was sleeping with his eyes closed. I wept and soon Ava was crying too. We left the room and soon they took his body away. My other sister Penny was there with her husband. My mother wanted to plan the memorial service and take care of the details right away.

I had some delusions around his death. I thought he knew he was going to die because I had warned him previously based on my clairvoyant abilities. I had recently given him a book to read by a certain bestseller author that I found in a shopping cart outside a store. So in my delusion, I believed that when I gave him the book by this author and when my older sister was pregnant with her next child, he would die. I told him to look for those signs. There's no proof of these predictions but rather I made a false connection between the present and past because of stress and grief.

During his lifetime, he did a lot of community service. Three months before he died, in a ceremony in Ottawa, the Prior of St. John knighted him for outstanding service.

At his memorial service, about five hundred people

attended. There were so many people; they couldn't fit in the sanctuary.

The family closed down his office. He had worked until the day before he died. At times, I feel he's still with me, watching over my life and thinking of me.

Writing, Art, and Public Speaking

June 2005 - April 2010

I wrote articles about the challenges of living with mental illness for *The Bulletin*, a mental health magazine. Reproduced images of my paintings were also included in their quarterly publication. It was a great opportunity to share my experiences and help others through writing.

Some people have a natural gift to write lyrical prose or rhythmic poetry. I was one of those who had to really work to achieve quality in writing. I wrote because I felt I had something to say and enjoyed the process.

I joined writers' forums on the Internet, to workshop screenplays, stories and poetry. I posted some of my writing. The reviewers were all members who could also submit their own work for review as well.

I made connections with other writers and we supported and motivated each other, giving feedback and sharing successes. For a year, I volunteered as a columnist for an online newsletter for one forum. Being a columnist improved my writing a great deal. I gained support from other writers. Eventually, I became the editor of the newsletter.

#

Over the years, I exhibited my art sporadically at restaurants, galleries, and other venues. I had some limited success in selling my work, but received many compliments on my sense of color and developing style.

As I moved along the road to wellness and better mental health, my art reflected my changing perceptions, and psychological and emotional state. I explored different genres including flowers, animals, surrealism and landscape. Also I began to see technical progress in my work. I improved my skills in color mixing, depth and form.

One friend said, "I think you are much happier now. I can see it in your paintings. You've come so far."

"Even though your subject matter changes, I can still identify your style. Your paintings are unique," another family friend said to me.

I took their comments to heart this time. I held on to the feeling upon hearing these compliments. I learned to accept praise from others.

A rehabilitation assistant at The Art Studios offered to curate a group show. She asked two others and me to give some samples of our work that we'd like to show. She successfully obtained a show at Gallery Gachet for us.

I wanted to keep to one genre this time. The show was called "Life Ineffable," meaning the unspoken, the taboo or the indescribable. I decided to use driftwood as the theme. How did driftwood relate to the ineffable? Here is an excerpt from my artist's statement:

Sandra begins with images and textures of driftwood and forms semi-abstract works that are indefinable. They are not totally representational or totally abstract but somewhere in between, acting on visual, mental, emotional, and metaphysical levels. As a person with a mental illness, her art reflects the dichotomy of her thought processes that are in constant flux.

Her interest in art started at a young age. The same hyperactivity and sensitivity that fueled her mental illness also led her to be an artist and a writer.

Why does she paint? She states it's a part of her yearning to escape and come alive on canvas. Her works contain traces of her essence.

#

After I quit work and attended classes at The Art Studios, I spent more time painting. During open studio, other talented artists would give me constructive feedback on my work. Greg told me my art became more consistent in quality. Instead of hits and misses, my work reached a new level.

One afternoon, my cousin and I went for a walk along the seawall. "I wish I was a famous artist," I said.

"When will you become famous?" she asked.

"Maybe when I'm dead." We laughed and gazed out at English Bay while sitting on a bench at Vanier Park. "But I wouldn't count on it."

"What makes you a good artist?"

"Perseverance, a bit of talent and the hope that I can reach my potential in art. Do you think I'm foolish to try? Would it be better to find a stable job that pays well so I can afford things?"

"You are living the dream of being an artist. Isn't that more important? Our other cousins can't write and paint like you."

I reflected on our conversation later. People perceived me as an artist and a writer. They appreciated my abilities. One woman at the studio referred to me as a "professional artist." That was significant that someone would think of me that way.

In the art world, there are the commercial artists who

make a living, the fine artists who struggle, and the Sunday painters who view art as leisure. I was a combination. I wanted to sell my art, I struggled, and I painted on Sundays!

In the whole world of art, I searched to find my niche. What made my art forgettable or unforgettable? How could I stand out in the crowd? Even if I never sold a painting for a thousand dollars or more, would I be content to know I had achieved integrity and quality in my art?

If artists were placed on a scale, I would be comfortably somewhere in the middle. I no longer strived to the best. I judged my paintings against others to understand my strengths and weaknesses as an artist. I saw my art more objectively. I once was very attached to my art and took any criticism personally. I had to separate the product - art or writing - from me as a person. Criticism of my work was not criticism of me, but something I made which I could improve. To think everything I created was a masterpiece was unrealistic.

Greg said, "Art comes from within you. It helps you. Any monies you make from selling art or writing is secondary, because you create to feel better."

It was a comfort to say art and writing were therapeutic but I wanted more. I wanted to take my art more seriously which meant I desired to exhibit and sell my work. Again, my ambitious nature rose inside of me. I was frustrated when I didn't sell work.

Soon I realized art could be appreciated without payment. I received a lot of good comments from people who saw my art through the Traveling Art Show. Similarly, I wanted to market my writing but success didn't happen overnight.

Dr. Sterling gave me some advice in regards to the times I felt I was stagnating. "Record good experiences in a journal, so that when you are discouraged or depressed you can look at it and remember those times."

I kept a journal of positive things that happened to me and another journal of negative thoughts that disturbed me. Later, I threw out the negative journal and kept the positive one.

#

Someone told me about the Wellness Recovery Action Plan (WRAP), a series of workshops, designed by Dr. Mary Ellen Copeland, an author, educator and advocate for mental health recovery. She also dealt with mental health difficulties.

I signed up to take WRAP led by two women who had taken the class previously and were certified as instructors. Each member of the group put together a book. Inside, I wrote a statement about my values and codes to live by. Sometimes I lost sight of my direction and goals and obsessed about things. I desired to be in control of my thoughts and feelings and enjoy my days in small ways. I chose to not depend on constant verbal approval from others to feel good self-esteem and try to build my own confidence from the inside out. I learned to do things in moderation.

I made a list of wellness tools including things or activities that made me feel good like mementos, humor, listening to music, watching movies, or going for coffee with friends. One important tool was to check the validity of negative thoughts or attitudes.

For example, I'd be suspicious that a friend was gossiping about me. First I asked myself, is this negative thought true? I needed to have a reality check. Sometimes I asked Greg and he would deny that the thought was true. Sometimes I believed him but other times I didn't. I looked for other signs to indicate if such ideas were symptoms or reality.

In one section of my WRAP book, I listed triggers that can bring on symptoms such as a change in the weather, stress, overdoing it, tiredness, spending too much time on the computer, or skipping a meal. My internal responses to these triggers were irritation, depression, self-doubt, worry, and tension.

If I spotted a trigger early, it was easier to remedy. I changed my activity, used self-talk, ate a snack, or found ways to relax. Sometimes I'd curl up on my bed in a dark room without stimuli.

Sometimes I couldn't identify an external trigger but I had psychotic symptoms of suspicion, clairvoyant experiences or grandiose ideas. These symptoms were followed by anxiety, an increase in obsessive thinking, fixation, agitation, loss of reality, talking to myself, or hostile rants.

Because my mind couldn't always think logically, it was very difficult to identify false ideas because I also depended on my mind for perception and objectivity. I looked for a pattern. I attempted to correct my mental distortions and get back on track. By labeling thoughts as symptoms not as reality, I distanced them and stopped them from controlling me.

Another workshop I found useful was Building

Recovery of Individual Dreams and Goals through Education and Support (BRIDGES). I learned about other mental illnesses and other strategies to keep well.

#

Prior to 2006, I was invited to talk to group home workers about challenges around providing care to mentally ill persons. The day I was to speak, I had a cough and itchy throat, which caused me some anxiety. I spoke loudly and made eye contact. I read from typed pages I had prepared. The audience listened closely. They asked me some questions.

"How do you get clients to exercise?" asked one participant. "I took a client swimming and he was fine, but when I asked him to go again, he repeatedly refused. What should I do?"

"There could be other issues around swimming that the client is uneasy about," I replied. "It takes a lot of effort to take the bus, get changed and swim for half an hour if one's out of shape or feels bad about their body image. Swimming can be tiring. The fact he went once was a good experience, but maybe you could try a different activity. Do you buy groceries as a group? Can you try going for coffee or cycling? Ask your client what he'd like to do."

"Thanks, that's good advice."

"We have clients that would really benefit from hearing you speak," said a female participant. "Many of our clients don't feel they can have a relationship but you're married. I think that would really mean a lot for them to hear from you."

#

I was invited to speak about recovery at two

187

Vancouver Community Mental Health Services orientations for staff and students. Some of the people asked me questions or said that they enjoyed hearing my talk.

One participant said, "I'm at a mental health team and have a client who has no family support and lives in a neighborhood where he is exposed to drug dealers. He comes to see me, but I don't know if I'm getting through to him. Do you have any suggestions for me about how to deal with him?"

"Ask him how he feels about the meetings you have," I replied. "The fact he is coming to your team means he is getting something out of it otherwise he wouldn't show. Make sure you tell him that marijuana or drug use can worsen mental illness in the long term. Truthfully, if he isn't supported by his family and is subjected to peer pressure, you may be the only lifeline he has. You are making a difference, whether you know it or not."

A nurse approached me during the break. "I've been rejected from employment in the mental health field because I have bipolar disorder."

"Despite how far we've come, there's still stigma in the system. I empathize. Because you have experienced illness, I would think you would be an employee of choice because you've lived it. I think the problem is employers in the mental health field or any field related to health want to protect themselves. If they feel an employee is not well, they may fear it will have an adverse effect on patients."

"I understand that all too well, but it's maddening that I'm judged on that criterion."

I had some good dialogue with people and the presenters. One woman told me, "You are a natural speaker. You listen to others' responses and incorporate that into your own talk."

One of the organizers who worked in family support asked what I would say to caregivers or families of mentally ill persons.

After I went home, I thought about it and wrote down ten suggestions for caregivers, which I will summarize here:

It's important to recognize the mentally ill person as an individual with unique abilities and strengths. Consumers want to be treated with respect. ("Consumer" is a term meaning receiver of services, patient or client. I only use it here as an abbreviation for persons with mental illness.)

Recognize and celebrate big and small successes of consumers. This may build their self-esteem. Watch out for changes in the consumer's behavior like depression or thought disturbance. Encourage the consumer to speak to his or her psychiatrist or mental health worker when issues come up. Keep the stress level low in the home if possible. If the consumer is feeling anxiety, suggest exercise, deep breathing or rest. If needed, encourage the person to take prescribed medication responsibly, eat a proper diet, and practice good hygiene. However, he or she may not like to be told.

By educating oneself about mental illness, one gains understanding and tolerance when a consumer behaves irrationally. Avoid confrontation. It's best to respond with forgiveness and compassion. Take breaks to keep yourself well in order to help the other person. Recognize one's efforts may contribute a lot to the well-being of the consumer.

For parents or spouses of mentally ill persons, they may spend a lot of time in a caregiver role, which can be draining and frustrating. Most learn by firsthand experience. Psychiatrists get paid, but caregivers don't get much.

Some consumers live alone but still depend on parents or siblings to aid them in grocery shopping or other tasks. Finances may be tight because the mentally ill person may have difficulty maintaining a job.

Another way families can help their loved ones is to advocate for consumer rights, more family involvement in care, housing, better community supports, and funding for research.

I emailed the ten points to the organizer. He emailed me back to ask if he could email my suggestions to his network of families. I agreed and felt glad that I could help others.

#

I was invited to speak at "Sharing our Success Stories" which consisted of panels of consumers speaking about art, education and volunteering. I spoke about the healing power of creating art to a group of consumers and family members of ill persons. It went very well. They applauded my story and made me feel recognized and proud of myself. Later, the organizers arranged a videotaping of four of us demonstrating our art skills and talking about the positive impact of creativity and art in our lives.

I got an email from the Vancouver/Richmond Regional Coordinator from the British Columbia

Schizophrenia Society (BCSS). She asked me if I was interested in giving a talk about my recovery to a high school class. I agreed.

At the talk, she spoke first about general information about schizophrenia. I listened to her talk about the causes and prevalence of schizophrenia.

"The current theory is that schizophrenia may be caused by a genetic predisposition combined with environmental stressors which trigger the onset of the illness. Other possible causes are being examined, including viruses during pregnancy, or problems during the birthing process.

"Schizophrenia affects one in a hundred of the population worldwide, spread equally across all ethnic groups. It affects men and women equally. The onset of schizophrenia is usually between the ages of fourteen and twenty-five but some can become ill in their thirties. If an individual has a schizophrenic disorder, the probability of a family member developing schizophrenia may depend on the amount of genes shared with that person. The closer one is related, the higher the probability. For example, if one identical twin develops schizophrenia, the other twin has a forty-eight percent chance of becoming ill. If a parent or other sibling has it, a person has a ten percent chance of developing schizophrenia."

After she spoke, I spoke about my recovery. When I finished, they clapped, which made me smile.

"What caused your illness? Was it genetic?" asked one student.

"I don't know of any family members who had schizophrenia. The doctors told me that I had a genetic vulnerability. Biological changes in puberty and stress in my environment triggered my illness."

Through the BCSS and networking, I had opportunities to speak about recovery to high school, college, and university students in various disciplines.

At various talks, I heard family members speak about difficulties dealing with a mentally ill spouse, son or daughter. They felt frustrated with the health system and lack of affordable housing. They wanted inclusion in the care of their loved ones but mental health professionals obeyed a code of doctor/patient confidentiality. Some patients didn't trust their families and requested no information on their case should be given to family. Some parents volunteered information to their loved one's psychiatrist, but it wasn't always a two-way street.

I heard family members speak about the pain of seeing their loved one suffer. Some mentally ill persons harm themselves. Some had concurrent disorders including substance abuse and a mental illness. Sometimes parents would get calls to pick up their adult child from emergency hospital services.

I felt deeply for the parents that shared their stories. They loved their children and recognized their strengths. It made me think more about the impact my illness and behaviors had on my family in the past and Greg in the present.

Giving talks gave me confidence because of the positive feedback I received. When I looked in the mirror, I no longer saw myself as a liability to society. Previously, I wanted to accomplish things in order to gain self-respect and self-esteem. I spent years trying to fit in, to live the life of a so-called normal person by attempting to work full-time and focus on a career that made me self-sufficient. But I discovered in the long run I couldn't keep up. The stress of work was too high and made me susceptible to symptoms despite regular use of medication.

I discovered I had a skill in public speaking and opportunity to encourage others. Instead of my needing attention and help, I could give compassion and insight to those who had similar experiences with mental illness and their families. When I spoke to families about my own journey of recovery, I think it gave them hope that their children could have quality of life.

Besides public speaking, I also have experience as a liaison worker for the Consumer Initiative Fund, a government-funded organization that offers educational and leisure activities for people with mental illness. The programs are peer-run, meaning the facilitators also have a mental illness. In this job, I learned better stress management, leadership, and assertiveness skills. I became more confident and found a sense of community there.

I was asked to co-lead a program evaluation of The Art Studios as a consumer voice. A PhD student and I designed and led focus groups. In 2009, the coordinator of the program, the PhD student, and I presented our findings at a Canadian Association of Occupational Therapists conference in Ottawa. I spoke about the program evaluation and gave my personal story including the ways being a member of The Art Studios had aided my recovery.

#

My life was like a traveling bus, making stops to drop off outdated assumptions and painful memories, and picking up new insights and opportunities. Since I began the recovery process, I experienced many epiphanies, many moments of discovery and insight. I continually learned and relearned along a winding road.

At a pivotal moment, I was having lunch with a relative and her two young children. I was complaining about my situation and how my illness held me back. She said, "Everyone experiences problems in their life. What you do with your life is your choice."

I realized that anyone, ill or not, has his or her own trials. It could be financial, social, psychological or plain bad luck. Life isn't perfect for anyone but the way one handles it is more important. I desired to remove the mental blocks that prevented me from moving forward and to rise to new challenges.

Ava invited me for a sushi lunch. "You know, our family doesn't think of you as the mentally ill one," she said. "We regard you as the creative one. You exceed limitations and overcome enormous obstacles in your life. I don't understand why you don't see it. I think you are a genius in the way you handle situations and take charge of your life. Hurray for you!"

Sitting at the restaurant, I remembered to hold onto those words and like myself instead of feeling self-pity as I had in the past. Once again, I had to let go of past barriers and be happy in the present.

In a discussion I had with Kathy, she said, "Be content with the here and now. Life isn't about achieving everything today. Be patient and enjoy the journey. You may get to the place you want to be in the future but it may not happen right away. I think you will reach some of your goals but be your own best friend. Celebrate the successes but be kind to yourself when you feel let down."

One friend suggested, "Reflect on the day before going to sleep and think about the positive things that happened that day or plan things you want to do for tomorrow. Reflection can help you to appreciate life with its ups and downs."

Having friends made a huge difference. Years ago, I had no close friends outside the family. Today I have several friends I can count on. I share more time with others and gain insights into how others handle crises. I can give and receive from others.

Gradually, I gained a better understanding. I think I'm finally getting my answers to lifelong questions. I've matured, learning to roll with the punches and accept myself, my talents and also my weaknesses, embracing my humanity. I see myself as a sum of parts.

I asked Greg, "Why have you stayed with me through so many years of outbursts and emotional distress on my part?"

He said, "There must be something about you more important or appealing than your upsets and problems. They are more minor than you think."

Later, in a moment of contemplation, I realized my tendency to exaggerate my problems. Greg and others saw the good in me.

#

I spent less time faultfinding. When I fell into that pattern, I realized the mechanism behind the behavior was built on my own insecurity.

I grew up. I no longer clung to the idea of being the

center of the world. I was more conscious of the line between reality and false beliefs. When stressed, I tried to act with reason and not react impulsively. When I experienced anger or hysteria, I bounced back.

In therapy sessions with Kathy, she was able to help me see my life more clearly and ease my doubts.

Dr. Sterling and I developed a rapport. He spoke more and I listened better and absorbed his suggestions and observations. Before I wasn't ready to hear him, but I became less rigid through therapy. I smiled, laughed and made bad puns.

Dr. Sterling seemed happier too. I'm not sure if the shift I saw in him was a sign of his own contentment or if he was responding to my new openness. He was proud of me. He said that I was a star client, articulate, intelligent, and charming.

I made a comment that my art wasn't marketable and thus I wasn't a successful artist.

He turned to me and said, "Believe me, you're big. You're a big artist."

I no longer have visits with Dr. Sterling because I was transferred to another mental health team. My new psychiatrist is also proactive in my care and encourages me a great deal.

He believes in me.

Stigma

To be honest, I've been fortunate enough not to experience much prejudice from others based on my illness. Sometimes the mentally ill can be the target of ridicule and abuse. It can be difficult to find employment or volunteer work if one reveals one has a mental illness. At times, the media describes the mentally ill as violent and aggressive but most aren't.

Stigma may not be obvious but implied like a murmur, a look of disdain, or a sarcastic remark. Sometimes ridicule can come from family or acquaintances who fear or don't understand the illness. When one experiences stigma, it hurts. It may cause anger, fear, or shame.

Sometimes people think if one is mentally ill, one has below average intelligence. They treat the person like a child or in a condescending manner. Some employers or volunteer coordinators may want to check with the consumer's doctor to confirm that the person will not act violently.

Even highly trained police officers may not be able to differentiate between a malicious person and someone who is acting erratically because they are mentally ill.

If a mentally ill person is hearing voices and disoriented, he or she may become fearful. If emergency is called with a complaint about a public disturbance, the situation must be handled skillfully. Police officers who use forced entry and enter a home with guns cocked may cause adverse reactions from a mentally ill person.

If I am a victim of stigma, I may choose to ignore it

or address the person who is expressing it. I could say that this is the behavior I observed and this is how it made me feel. For example, I could say, "I don't like the use of the words 'mental case' or 'psycho.' It made me feel angry."

It takes courage but if I can stand up for myself, I gain dignity and the other person is made aware of their error. The next time that person makes a crack about a "crazy nutcase" neighbor, he or she may think twice.

I believe in having a fair community without stigma. For me, raising awareness begins with conversing with people I know personally. Talking and writing about mental health issues reduces preconceptions. If others can accept me or put a face to schizophrenia, their view of mental illness may change.

I hope that issues around stigma can change for the better. I desire to do my part by speaking up and staying informed of government policy, social programs and opportunities for the mentally ill.

#

My experience with stigma came mainly from inside myself. When I had my first psychotic episode, it hit me hard because I already lacked self-confidence and was too young to really understand.

I believed I had brought the illness on myself. I searched for reasons for my suffering, but couldn't find them. I had a lot of negative self-talk. I considered myself an outcast. I withdrew and minimized contact with other people. I stopped caring about myself. Self-stigma robbed me of feeling self-worth. I thought I was a weak person.

The question is then, how did I recover from my loss of self?

On a trip to Italy, I saw the statue of David in Florence. It was magnificent. When Michelangelo sculpted David, he spent over three years of careful attention to chip away and polish it until he perfected it. He started with a block of marble that transformed into one of the most highly regarded sculptures in history.

I thought about Michelangelo's long hours creating this piece of art. He believed that the image of David was already in the stone waiting to be revealed. In a way, I was carving my own sculpture. Over a period of many years, slowly I peeled away a rough, weathered external shell, reached into my soul and found myself. I wasn't the statue of David, but I was uniquely me.

I gained a new identity. I saw myself as a human being first, a writer and an artist but also a productive contributor to society. I was engaged with the outside world. I also had the roles of daughter, sister, niece, spouse, friend, sister-in-law, and aunt.

As I matured, I developed a more objective view of the way I fit into the world. Instead of regarding my chronic illness as a punishment, I accepted it.

I reduced negative self-talk and accepted positive reinforcement from others. Believing in myself was the beginning of the process. I reflected on my development as a person. Communicating with others broadened my perspective. Seeing myself the way others did, was an eye-opener. At The Art Studios and when presenting talks to students, I felt respected. When I spoke about my recovery, I was applauded.

In the face of stigma, I needed to feel centered and balanced within myself. Purpose kept me from focusing on my problems and boosted my self-esteem. Meaningful work, paid or unpaid, and leisure activities gave me a feeling of accomplishment and enjoyment.

I recognized my identity wasn't determined by my illness. There was more to me than a diagnosis.

Reflections

In the past few years, I think some misconceptions have lessened because of awareness, education, early psychosis intervention and scientific research. Today schizophrenia is regarded as a brain disease, which eliminates some misunderstanding about the illness. Schizophrenia is not a split personality but defined as a split with reality.

The British Columbia mental health system has changed dramatically. Previously, care for the mentally ill was based on the traditional model of treating the illness through medication and electroconvulsive therapy and not treating the person as a whole.

Deinstitutionalization in the late 80's to 90's in Vancouver and its surrounding area, more specifically the downsizing of Riverview Hospital in Coquitlam, put vulnerable people on the street without community support. More recently, the government is attempting to supply more shelters and housing for the homeless, including the mentally ill.

Health workers are more pro-active in the care of their clients. As part of psychosocial rehabilitation, occupational therapists and other people in the mental health field use programs and activities to aid clients in finding purposeful work, educational, leisure or volunteer pursuits.

Despite problems in the system because of politics or lack of funding, overall I think mental health providers in B.C. do the best they can with the tools they have. I believe their intentions are good even if they make mistakes. That's my experience; everyone's story is different.

For the mentally ill, hope is crucial for building motivation and determination. One needs to be adaptable to situations, taking into account personal strengths, limitations and external barriers. Having purpose and satisfaction in one's daily activities builds self-worth and value.

Consumers have unique experiences, emotional and psychological make-up, and brain chemistry, and thus require different combinations of medications and different solutions to the problems they face. Setting goals and taking on new challenges depends on the readiness and confidence of the individual.

So what can the mentally ill do well? They can crack jokes about mental illness and the system. Many have creative ability. They respond to the right type of care and therapy. They smile when someone recognizes them for who they are. They can aid each other because they've suffered in similar ways and dealt with similar issues. They are heroes to me because they deal with issues everyday. For some, their lives are a constant battle to keep themselves well.

I think it's important that clients have a voice about innovations and programs in mental health services. By working together with families and mental health providers, they can effect change in the system for the better.

There's a saying, "If you haven't got your health, you haven't got anything."

Wellness is about how we live day by day and survive in a turbulent world, and that goes for anyone not just the mentally ill.

Recovery doesn't always mean being cured and not needing medication. It means having a fulfilling life, self-acceptance, and social inclusion.

What makes recovery possible? In my case, I have the care and stability of a good home where I'm expected to act responsibly and reasonably. My family sees through my illness to Sandra, the real me. Others believe in me and help me develop tools to build a better life.

I have no history of alcohol or drug abuse. I take my medicine as prescribed because I know it helps me function better. I'm not immune to conflicts and stress that are part of everyday life.

I remember walking around with a cloud over my head that rained on me for years like in a cartoon. Since then, I've built myself an umbrella of hope. Now the sun has come out and the sky is clear. I don't fear rainy days because the sun will come out again tomorrow. There's a part of me that believes change is possible, and that is the great hope that pushes me forward.

Good insight is key to my mental wellness. I am healthier emotionally and psychologically, because I can recognize triggers and take precautions to keep myself well. I have a sense of self-worth.

I am motivated and determined to work through difficulties and meet challenges. Without direction and initiative, I would be lost.

I know other consumers who are in recovery and have quality of life. They socialize and maintain friendships and relationships. They enjoy a sense of balance in their leisure occupations. They benefit from the right medications and care from psychiatrists and mental health teams. Some are well enough to be employed, go to school or volunteer. Some are peer support workers who help others.

Anyone can have a bad day or week when things aren't going right and react in different ways. Many have dysfunction in their relationships, problems in the past, or difficulty coping in their lives at various times. Society determines who fits into the norm of acceptable behavior. Everyone struggles with some issue or setback. We adapt and hopefully we overcome.

#

I went for an evening walk in my neighborhood, taking photos of flowers, trees, picket fences and picturesque houses. A row of tall Douglas firs cast long shadows across the grass. I sat outside, watching the change in light as the sun descended in the sky. The sweet scent of honeysuckle filled the air. I smelled smoke from meat grilling on a neighbor's barbeque. Crows called from the trees.

I looked through the lens of my camera. A ring of light created a halo around the sun. I blinked and the halo disappeared. Were my eyes playing tricks on me? Did the camera allow me to see things beyond objective reality? I took another picture. This time the sky was pink and mauve. Cumulus clouds caught the light. It was getting darker. I held the camera as steadily as I could and took more shots.

Sometimes when taking pictures, the things I focused on weren't the same as other people. Others would see only greenery, but I saw layers of grass, leaves and ferns with individual characteristics. I took many photos of the same thing over and over until I got the shot I wanted.

In the cool breeze, I closed my eyes. I imagined myself floating in the air. I felt a sense of peace, free of disturbing thoughts. Slowly, the sun disappeared behind the roofs and fences. In the brief silence, I was alone.

I preferred pictures of nature to photos of myself. Those were much more acceptable, not reflecting the internal self but the external world.

We've heard the saying, "The camera doesn't lie." However, the things I chose to see or not see in life frame my reality. Sometimes I got caught up in the details and didn't see the larger picture.

I decided my illness wasn't a life sentence. I found the silver lining to my illness.

I learned the value of my family and friends who stood by me at different times in my life. I was treated with kindness and compassion.

I learned to respect myself and see myself honestly. Instead of being driven and narrow in my viewpoint, I try to see things in a broader context. Therapy helped me to develop better problem-solving techniques and insight into my personality.

I took the time to develop my art and writing. I believed the elevated states of hypomania related to illness were linked to my exaggerated imagination and creative ability to write, paint and draw.

I have a support network of friends, co-workers and family. I reciprocate the care I've received by reaching out to others. I accept who I am, and I value my life, despite struggle and loss.

I hope reading this true account has given you insight into the barriers of mental illness and a personal journey of recovery. This story is finished up to this point in my life, but I hope in the future I will have many more stories to tell.

Biography

Sandra has a Fine Arts Diploma from Langara College in Vancouver and a Bachelor of Arts degree from the University of British Columbia, majoring in art history. She is an artist and exhibits her colorful acrylic paintings locally.

Her articles, stories and poems have appeared in *Front Magazine, The Bulletin, The Prairie Journal,* and other print and online publications.

She has given numerous talks about her recovery to mental health consumers, families, high school, college and university students, and mental health professionals. Some of her speaking engagements have been through the British Columbia Schizophrenia Society.

She worked jointly on a program evaluation of The Art Studios (a program which offers classes in the creative arts to people with mental health conditions) and helped to organize and co-lead focus groups. As a result, she jointly published an article on collaborative practice between occupational therapists and mental health consumers, which appeared in the *PSR/RPS Express* newsletter in the fall of 2008. She spoke at the 2009 Canadian Association of Occupational Therapists Conference about the program evaluation and the benefits of the program in her own recovery.

In the past, she taught creative writing. She has experience as a liaison worker for the Consumer Initiative Fund, which offers peer-run leisure and educational activities for people with mental illness. She also has experience as a columnist and editor for *Majestic,* an online newsletter for Lit.org, an online writers' forum.

Sandra believes strongly in reducing stigma and building awareness of mental illness.

OTHER SIMILAR TITLES FROM BRIDGEROSS

The Adolescent Owner's Manual by David Laing Dawson MD. 978-0-9866522-0-2, 2010, 154 pages, $15.95, distributed by Ingram and QBI

A refreshing look at the puzzling world faced by today's teens and the moms and dads who are trying to guide them. Incorporating advances in neuroscience, psychiatrist David Dawson clearly describes how teen brains work and offers practical advice to baffled parents in a fun and relaxing style.

After Her Brain Broke: Helping My Daughter Recover Her Sanity, by Susan Inman 978-0-9810037-8-8, 2010, 168 pages, $18.95, distributed by Ingram.

"A model for other families. Highly recommended" Dr. E Fuller Torrey, author of *Surviving Schizophrenia* and former advisor to the National Alliance For the Mentally Ill.

Schizophrenia: Medicine's Mystery Society's Shame, by Marvin Ross, 978-0-9810037-0-2, 2008, 188 pages, $19.95, distributed by Ingram and QBI

"a powerful resource for anyone looking for answers and insight into the world of mental illness." Schizophrenia Digest Magazine.

The Brush, The Pen and Recovery, A 33 minute documentary on schizophrenia distributed by Moving Images, Vancouver, BC "profoundly moving, educational and hopeful." Eufemia Fanteti author and performer of "My Own Private Etobicoke", Toronto, ON .

LaVergne, TN USA
29 October 2010

202715LV00005B/206/P